What doctors don't know
about you can cost money,
illness, your life. Keep
separate records for every
member of your family in his
or her own copy of

Your Lifetime Health Records Book

Health Records of

(name of individual)

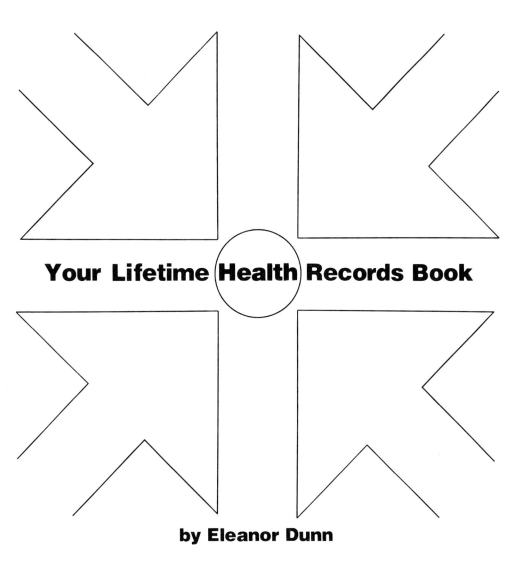

Your Lifetime Health Records Book

by Eleanor Dunn

McGRAW-HILL BOOK COMPANY
New York   St. Louis   San Francisco   Düsseldorf
Mexico   Toronto

Book design by Morris Kirchoff.

123456789RABP79876

Library of Congress Cataloging in Publication Data

Dunn, Eleanor, date
    Your lifetime health records book.

        1.   Medical records. 2.   Medicine, Popular.
I.   Title.
R864.D86   613   75-31870
ISBN 0-07-018271-X

Plates showing "Skeleton and Skull," "Viscera," "Muscles," and "Eye"
originally appeared in *Blakiston's Gould Medical Dictionary,* 3rd. ed.,
edited by A. Osol and C. C. Francis, copyright © 1972 by McGraw-Hill,
Inc. Used by permission of McGraw-Hill Book Company.

Where are your health records now?

Scattered. On scraps of paper that get lost. In an older relative's memory. Hidden in files wherever you have received health care. Lost or destroyed over the years.

Doctors deplore the lack of records on patients, but they can't take time to dig up data from previous doctors and hospitals or to organize facts in sequences to be significant. It is *your* health. It is up to you to find out and keep your own vital records to show every physician and specialist who cares for you during your lifetime.

Doctors have a vast store of knowledge, but what doctors don't know about *you* can include your particular drug allergies, genetic tendencies, immunizations, previous disorders, results of diagnostic tests, other doctors' concurrent therapy, and additional facts that will fill this book. Only after they know your individual health records can they do their best in diagnosing and treating you as an individual. Except for communicable diseases, an illness doesn't happen suddenly. It builds up with blood pressure and cholesterol levels, for instance.

Good health care requires the cooperation of patient with doctor and of doctors with doctors. You are one total living being who cannot be treated in pieces. A disorder in one part of your body can disturb other parts. A drug given by one doctor may alter the effect of a drug given by another doctor. Unknown facts can cause needless problems.

This book does not present diagnoses or therapy for diseases. Only a doctor can determine those, after he or she knows your health records and examines you and after he or she has results of any needed tests.

This book offers a convenient means of communication and cooperation between you and your doctors that has never before been available. It presents orderly places to keep data which doctors can find quickly by checking the table of contents. Because you are the one who decides when to see a doctor, it gives you condensed information on the body and some signs and symptoms that should alert you to see a physician or dentist promptly.

It identifies the most frequent diagnostic procedures, helps you decide when you can (or dare not) save on medical costs, helps you analyze health insurance policies, explains prescriptions and drug interactions, suggests how you can help trace allergies, relieve stress, care for your teeth and skin, and tend to common disorders. And it gives other information because what *you* don't know about health can also cost money, illness, your life.

The book takes a realistic look at the American health care system which has been called "sick," more by professionals who know it well than by the public. This is not a perfect world. Should perfection be expected only in the medical and dental professions? However, improvements can be made by both doctors and patients, and this book points out a few.

The big problem has been too little information with subsequent lack of understanding and appreciation of other viewpoints. When information is disclosed, perhaps there can be more cooperation in preventing and fighting disease. That's the only purpose of health care. The virtual eradication of polio, smallpox, and tuberculosis shows what can be done. Decreasing disease rates should be the constructive concern of all patients, as well as all doctors and everyone else in the giant health care industry. The professionals are outnumbered by the patients, so much of the task must be the public's. If each person knew his or her individual health condition, what to guard against, and what to do to regain or maintain health, at least the intelligent and motivated ones would do much to improve their own health and the nation's health average.

This book is not "literature." It is an informative guide and organized record-keeper for use by you and your doctors. It does not pretend to cover all phases of health. Large libraries and 300 professional journals published each month can hardly do that. Statistics provided here are the most recent ones available at the time of writing and are given, along with a few actual case histories, to let you know of the need to be personally involved in your own health.

Because each person's health records are different, you will want a copy of this book for each member of your family. Start your children's books now to show health heritage, list health records while they are being made, and supply data that will be valuable throughout their lives.

Contents

Illustrations

(Include phone area codes and postal zip codes throughout records)

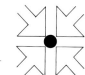

My name _____

Home address _____

City, State _____

Home phone _____ **Business phone** _____

Dr. _____

Office address _____

City, State _____

Office phone _____ **Home phone** _____

Emergency personnel need to know:

Speak English _____; **other languages** _____.

Deaf _____. **Blind** _____. **Mentally retarded** _____. **Scuba diver** _____.

Heart problem _____; **taking drug?** _____.

Wear pacemaker _____; **implanted?** _____. **Wear contact lenses** _____.

Diabetes _____; **on insulin?** _____. **Epilepsy** _____; **drug** _____.

Neck breather (after tracheostomy) _____. **Asthma** _____.

Glaucoma _____. **Hemophilia** _____.

Now taking anticoagulant _____; **cortisone** _____; **thyroid drug** _____.

Are you now pregnant? _____.

Other _____.

Blood type _____.

Allergic to: Penicillin _____. **Morphine** _____. **Tetanus serum** _____.

Sulfa _____. **Aspirin** _____. **Insect stings** _____.

Other relating to emergencies ___ _____.

Always wear an identification bracelet or neck tag if you have a rare blood type or any special problem that must be known in emergency situations. See "Checkpoints to Guard Your Health" in the following section of the book.

CURRENT IDENTIFICATION

Height _____

Weight _____

(Space for small picture of face)

Hair _____

Skin tone _____

Eye color _____

Glasses _____

Any identifying feature, birthmark, or scar _____

Hospital with my records _____

Street, City, State _____

Relative or friend _____

Home phone _____ Business phone _____

Relative or friend _____

Home phone _____ Business phone _____

Employed by _____

City, State _____ Phone _____

Employed by _____

City, State _____ Phone _____

Health insurance or HMO: See table of contents.

Medicare No. _____ Social Security No. _____

Keep information on these two pages up to date. If you expect to have frequent changes, use a pencil and erase. After a period of years, x out and fill in the next "Emergency?" pages. Do not tear out at binding.

10

(Include phone area codes and postal zip codes throughout records)

Emergency?

My name _____

Home address _____

City, State _____

Home phone _____ **Business phone** _____

Dr. _____

Office address _____

City, State _____

Office phone _____ **Home phone** _____

Emergency personnel need to know:

Speak English _____ ; **other languages** _____ .

Deaf _____ . **Blind** _____ . **Mentally retarded** _____ . **Scuba diver** _____ .

Heart problem _____ ; **taking drug?** _____ .

Wear pacemaker _____ ; **implanted?** _____ . **Wear contact lenses** _____ .

Diabetes _____ ; **on insulin?** _____ . **Epilepsy** _____ ; **drug** _____ .

Neck breather (after tracheostomy) _____ . **Asthma** _____ .

Glaucoma _____ . **Hemophilia** _____ .

Now taking anticoagulant _____ ; **cortisone** _____ ; **thyroid drug** _____ .

Are you now pregnant? _____ .

Other _____ .

Blood type _____ .

Allergic to: Penicillin _____ . **Morphine** _____ . **Tetanus serum** _____ .

       Sulfa _____ . **Aspirin** _____ . **Insect stings** _____ .

       Other relating to emergencies _____ .

Always wear an identification bracelet or neck tag if you have a rare blood type or any special problem that must be known in emergency situations. See "Checkpoints to Guard Your Health" in the following section of the book.

CURRENT IDENTIFICATION

Height _____

Weight _____

Hair _____

(Space for small
picture of face)

Skin tone _____

Eye color _____

Glasses _____

Any identifying feature, birthmark, or scar _____

Hospital with my records _____

Street, City, State _____

Relative or friend _____

Home phone _____ Business phone _____

Relative or friend _____

Home phone _____ Business phone _____

Employed by _____

City, State _____ Phone _____

Employed by _____

City, State _____ Phone _____

Health insurance or HMO: See table of contents.

Medicare No. _____ Social Security No. _____

Keep information on these two pages up to date. If you expect to have frequent changes, use a pencil and erase. After a period of years, x out and fill in the next "Emergency?" pages. Do not tear out at binding.

(Include phone area codes and postal zip codes throughout records)

Emergency?

My name _____

Home address _____

City, State _____

Home phone _____ **Business phone** _____

Dr. _____

Office address _____

City, State _____

Office phone _____ **Home phone** _____

Emergency personnel need to know:

Speak English _____ ; **other languages** _____ .

Deaf _____ . **Blind** _____ . **Mentally retarded** _____ . **Scuba diver** _____ .

Heart problem _____ ; **taking drug?** _____ .

Wear pacemaker _____ ; **implanted?** _____ . **Wear contact lenses** _____ .

Diabetes _____ ; **on insulin?** _____ . **Epilepsy** _____ ; **drug** _____ .

Neck breather (after tracheostomy) _____ . **Asthma** _____ .

Glaucoma _____ . **Hemophilia** _____ .

Now taking anticoagulant _____ ; **cortisone** _____ ; **thyroid drug** _____ .

Are you now pregnant? _____ .

Other _____ .

Blood type _____ .

Allergic to: Penicillin _____ . **Morphine** _____ . **Tetanus serum** _____ .

Sulfa _____ . **Aspirin** _____ . **Insect stings** _____ .

Other relating to emergencies _____ _____ .

Always wear an identification bracelet or neck tag if you have a rare blood type or any special problem that must be known in emergency situations. See "Checkpoints to Guard Your Health" in the following section of the book.

CURRENT IDENTIFICATION

Height _____

Weight _____

Hair _____   (Space for small
                                   picture of face)
Skin tone _____

Eye color _____

Glasses _____

Any identifying feature, birthmark, or scar _____

Hospital with my records _____

Street, City, State _____

Relative or friend _____

Home phone _____ Business phone _____

Relative or friend _____

Home phone _____ Business phone _____

Employed by _____

City, State _____ Phone _____

Employed by _____

City, State _____ Phone _____

Health insurance or HMO: See table of contents.

Medicare No. _____ Social Security No. _____

14

You move—an average of fourteen times during a lifetime. Every year one out of five Americans moves. In each new city or town your new doctors need your health history.

You are referred to specialists—but your comprehensive records stay in your primary physician's office. Each specialist does not take your complete health history. He or she diagnoses and treats disorders in part of your body, although the health of all parts is interrelated.

You travel—around the city and around the world. A temporary doctor needs to know about your immunizations, medications, allergies, or chronic diseases so he or she can give immediate treatment that is right for you. When you become ill in your home area, information included in this book names your doctors and the hospital which has data on your health.

If injured in an accident in an area where hospitals specialize in different types of emergency care, you will be taken to the one best equipped for your needs, not necessarily the nearest one or the one with your records. Paramedics on ambulances can transmit vital signs and health records via two-way radio to a hospital doctor who has never seen you but can direct the start of life-saving treatment at the site and en route to the emergency room.

If you check into a hospital on the advice of your doctor, you usually have time to go home and pack a bag. Make sure this book goes in along with your toothbrush.

In case you are attended by a foreign physician, show these records; 17 percent of all doctors in the United States are foreign-born. Accents and language barriers can hamper oral communication, but reading English is easier for them.

While under the stress of anxiety, severe pain, or fever, it is difficult to remember health facts. Both you and the doctor fret at the time it takes to ask and answer questions and for him to write out a patient history chart. But doctors need to know certain facts before they can give emergency relief or examine, diagnose, and prescribe for you.

With a glance at Contents and the pages in this record, a doctor could find out, for instance, that your immediate problem (called "presenting complaint") might stem from another disorder you have had. Looking at a page of sequential records on high blood pressure or test results, he or she can see the progress or the arresting of a chronic disorder. A doctor could write the desired information on your patient record chart while you are undressing for examination or giving samples of body fluids to technicians. The doctor's

You and Your Doctors Need Records for Better Health Care (Often at Lower Cost)

15

nurse-practitioner or certified aide could fill in other data while the doctor attends you.

Only 15 percent of all physicians are reported to be in general family practice. If you do not have a private physician but go to specialists, clinics, or hospital emergency rooms whenever you are sick, your book of health records is absolutely essential. No temporary doctor or specialist has time to trace your records. He will diagnose according to his findings at the time you see him. If tests are needed, it is faster to order new ones and ignore previous data except for what you can relate, often in less than five minutes. One examination and one set of tests seldom reveal conclusive evidence of a disease. You may not be treated for the disorder you have.

Fragments of your health records are in the offices of ophthalmologists, dentists, and podiatrists. In addition to diagnoses and therapy in their specialties, they can see in your eyes and mouth and on your feet possible disorders developing in other parts of your body—often before you notice specific symptoms. They could help you by calling your physician or suggesting you see him.

Doctors' Office Records

Considering there are about 10,000 known diseases and 100,000 observable findings in modern Western medicine, your doctors can use all the information they can get on their patients. Medical journals carry many articles and letters by doctors who feel frustrated by the lack of complete medical histories. Yet a doctor cannot delay diagnosis and therapy for an illness until widely scattered records are located. It is too time-consuming to try to obtain records from other doctors who may have moved, transferred your files to another doctor or basement storeroom, be at a convention or on vacation, or be much too busy to respond to a request for records on a former patient. Occasionally, records are destroyed in fire or lost during transport. This book assures another set.

Doctors' office records generally consist of (1) patient profile (name, address, age, occupation, marital status, health insurance company, referring doctor or patient), (2) data base (patient history, examination findings, reports on tests), (3) problem list which includes symptoms and diagnoses, (4) treatment sheet, and (5) progress notes.

Too often the printed form used during your initial visit is followed by plain, loose sheets with an assortment of scrawls made during each visit. There is no one place or chronological order for blood pressure readings, immunizations, disorders in each body system, etc. Laboratory reports are scattered among papers in the folder and can easily be lost. Phoned reports on electrodiagnoses may not be noted in your file.

With inadequate or no records, how is a doctor to remember every ailment of every patient? For example, a physician asked a patient whether she ever had a previous attack, although three years earlier he had admitted her to a hospital for diagnostic tests and treatment for the same disorder. And a pediatrician asked parents during every visit what immunizations she had given each child and when.

Reports on your X rays, electrocardiograms, laboratory tests, and other studies are the property of the doctor who ordered them made, though you paid for them. The doctor keeps these records for as long as he wishes (at most fifteen to twenty years) and then destroys them. If a doctor turns over a patient's records to another doctor, they become that doctor's property. Hospitals keep records "forever," transferring bulky ones like X rays to microfilm after a certain number of years which varies with hospitals.

Do You Have a Right to Know?

Consumer rights are increasing in most areas. The Freedom of Information Act made it legal for the public to obtain information from government employes who acquire information for public benefit. This applies to foods, drugs, product safety, food additives, pesticides, etc. Consumers have the right to know the contents of their files at credit bureaus.

For 200 years Americans have had the right to life, liberty, and the pursuit of happiness, but too many are still denied the right to health or to know about their health. In many states patients do not have a legal right to inspect or copy their own medical records. Doctors think patients will misinterpret what they read and become alarmed—and doctors don't have time to explain. Some states are changing laws to enable patients to obtain their records through lawyers, leaving it to a lawyer's discretion as to what information to disclose and expecting a lawyer to explain medical facts. The patient pays fees to the lawyer as well as the doctor.

The confidentiality of the doctor-patient relationship is

further broken by supplying information to (1) U.S. Public Health Service, (2) medical institutions which share patient information for research purposes, (3) technicians and office workers who obtain, record, file, and computerize data in the offices of doctors and the record rooms of hospitals and laboratories, (4) employers who see group health insurance claims, (5) health and life insurance companies. The Medical Information Bureau keeps records on medical ailments of the millions of individuals who have ever applied for life insurance. The pool is used by more than 700 insurance companies. Facts on applicants are given as guidelines for the companies' own investigations.

While there is no law requiring a doctor to give information to a patient, there is no law to prevent you from asking your doctor for clearly explained facts about your personal health, keeping your own health records, and asking the doctor to make entries. A patient need no longer be patient about the right to know.

More and more doctors are now giving facts to patients because they have found it gains patient cooperation. Most hospitals are recognizing patients' rights, encouraging doctors to inform their patients, and suggesting greater communication all around.

The American Hospital Association, an organization comprising about 7,000 institutional members and more than 20,000 personal members, approved *A Patient's Bill of Rights* in 1973. Its twelve provisions cover areas such as the following:

1. The patient has the right to considerate and respectful care.
2. The patient (or an appropriate person in his behalf) has the right to obtain from his physician complete current information concerning his diagnosis, treatment, and prognosis [the forecast of the probable course of a disease] in terms that can be understood.
3. The patient has the right to receive from his physician information necessary to give informed consent to the start of any procedure and/or treatment. Where medically significant alternatives exist, the patient has the right to such information.
4. The patient has the right to refuse treatment to the extent permitted by law, and to be informed of the medical consequences of his action.
5. The patient has the right to be advised if the hospital proposes to perform human experimentation affecting his care or treatment . . . and the right to refuse to participate in such research projects.

18

6. The patient has the right to examine and receive an explanation of his bill, regardless of the source of payment.*

Ask the Doctor—It's Your Health

If your doctor doesn't tell you freely, don't be afraid to ask about your condition and the findings of the physical examination and the various tests made. Why take the chance some people do—those who never ask their physicians why they aren't feeling well, saying they wouldn't understand medical language and don't want to take up the doctor's valuable time to explain?

The wife of one such man did ask their physician about her health after every checkup, kept records on her high blood pressure and high cholesterol levels, and adopted measures to reduce them. The doctor assumed the couple was on the same diet—but the husband, unaware he had the same problems, ate chocolate candy and added lots of salt and butter to the low-salt, low-fat meals his wife prepared. He was given no reason to take medication, so he did not have his prescription filled. He had a heart attack.

Patients pay over $8 billion a year for prescriptions, but millions of additional prescriptions are not filled. Many people relax after they have given the doctor their problems and money, feeling no need to spend more time and money at a pharmacy.

Rarely do patients have an opportunity to question medical authorities or dogma. Few doctors stray from "the usual and customary standards of medical practice," although some older practices may have been found ineffective or harmful since first accepted and some newer methods have been known to work for two decades. The feudal system in which doctors work and the Food and Drug Administration move slowly and not always surely. Another fifteen federal bureaus purport to help consumers, but many of their activities are on a trial-and-error basis.

Like freedom of speech, no one recognizes the value of health until it is lost. To assure the best possible health for yourself and your family, *you* need to become involved. Do you really believe "*They* will take care of my health," when "they" are humans, too? They get tired, have personal problems, make mistakes, want approval and recognition, and are annoyed by some patients.

*Adapted from *A Patient's Bill of Rights*, with the permission of the American Hospital Association.

On the other hand, doctors try to be always courteous and efficient. They say patients expect too much from them. They cannot guarantee results. Success rates vary with the nature of an illness, medical technology available, therapy used, possible unforeseen complications, the doctor's skill, and the patient's cooperation. Yet many patients expect miracles in every case and place their physicians on pedestals.

An old-fashioned posture, once taught in medical schools, is still assumed by some doctors. It gave the doctor the privilege of presenting a godlike authoritarian image and of merely telling the patient, "Don't worry—I'll watch out for your health." That may have served when patient and doctor lived in the same small town for the same long years of residence. The doctor knew the family's health, took time to teach health care, and saw the patient frequently around town as well as in the office.

In those days doctors dispensed more assurance than medications. They had no sophisticated diagnostic aids to help distinguish an ailment or "wonder drugs" to treat it. Today some physicians still do not take time to isolate a causative agent. It is easier to prescribe general (broad-spectrum) antibiotics with uncertain benefits and possible unwanted side effects than to find specific ills in order to give specific pills. (However, in emergencies and occasional cases, broad-spectrum drugs can be life-savers.)

The rapid advances in medical knowledge have made it impossible for any one physician or dentist to know everything. That is why intelligent people no longer rely on only one. They go to several specialists, each of whom should check records on the total patient before treating a part.

For the population as a whole, health and lifetime expectancies are improving. Major credit is due not only to improved medical care but also to Americans learning more about health and taking better care of themselves. Further gains can be made if everyone does more than simply complain that the sick care system in the United States is sick.

The distribution of health care is a big problem. Doctors prefer to practice where hospitals offer advanced medical technology, shunning country towns without facilities. Many prefer to live and work in wealthy suburbs near large medical centers. Doctors prefer to limit their numbers by not modernizing curricula and teaching and by not otherwise supporting medical schools. The need is greatest for general practitioners interested in disease prevention, which includes nutrition.

Some areas have one doctor in private practice for 600 to 1,000 people. In other sections this ratio may be one doctor for 4,000 to 10,000 people. Patients without access to a private physician must use municipal facilities, because it requires a doctor's orders for a patient to enter a private hospital or nursing home and to obtain outpatient diagnostic tests or prescriptions.

These are concerns for patients, doctors, hospitals, health insurance companies, and government agencies which help fund medical schools through research grants and could do more investigating of fraud and waste in government-sponsored programs for health and insurance, in nursing homes, and in environmental control.

The New Breed of Doctors

Since medicine is an art, not an exact science, doctors have differing opinions on virtually every subject. This includes attitudes to take toward patients. Some play a stern, patronizing role, expect patients to be passive and have blind faith, and tell them little or nothing. A doctor's innocent "Hmm," without explanation, has been known to make a patient afraid he had some awful disease.

Doctors of the new breed are working to overcome the conspiracy of silence that has long dominated the profession. As the president of a medical college said, "The days of great secrecy in medicine are long gone." Doctors who are wise in human relations recognize that an intelligent, emotionally stable patient who wants to know has the right to know about his diagnosis, therapy, and prognosis.

These compassionate doctors observe from a patient's eyes and tenseness when fear of the unknown is inducing his imagination to suspect the worst. Tension and anxiety do not promote healing. Relaxation and confidence in the doctor and therapy do. Information given promptly, kindly, and clearly often prevents or lessens hypochondria, undue anxiety about health. Anxiety creates more inner conflicts than actual neuroses caused by overaction of the nervous system, self-provoked or caused by an actual disease or injury.

When predictive tests indicate a patient may at some future time develop a disease, the doctor judges whether the particular individual may be harmed by worrying about something that may never happen or whether he should discuss the possibility and teach the patient health measures to help delay or prevent the condition from developing. If an illness may be terminal, the physician ascertains how much information an individual wants and can accept at the time. If any patient makes it clear that health facts would be distressing, the physician honors this feeling.

Occasionally, doctors may record in this book the medical terms which inform other doctors of the nature of an illness more precisely, though it's literally Greek to you. If you want to know, ask for simple English words.

When you see a physician, what easy-to-understand information should you expect? (1) Results of any diagnostic tests as soon as the doctor receives reports. "Negative" is good; it means the condition for which the test was made is not present. (2) What the ailment is. (3) How often and when to take prescribed medications. How they work and their possible side effects, such as drowsiness, headache, gastric discomfort. Whether alcohol, aspirin, antacids, antihistamines, or other over-the-counter (nonprescription) drugs will affect the action of his prescribed therapy. (4) How long recovery may take if there are no complications. (5) Whether you can help speed recovery with special diet, bed rest, exercise, hot or cold applications, no smoking, or whatever is relevant.

You have the right to receive a doctor's bill according to your agreement with him. This can be at the end of each visit, on a monthly, quarterly, or yearly basis, or submitted promptly for you to make an insurance claim, unless the physician sends the bill directly to your insurer. If you are a regular patient, you should be told if you will be charged for advice given over the phone.

Doctor-patient relationships have been strained by lack of understanding. Example: A patient who had twisted a foot met her physician in a hospital corridor. He glanced at but did not touch her foot and told his shadowing intern to have it X rayed. Six months after the hospital bill for X rays and report of no fractures was paid by the insurance company, she received a $25 bill from her doctor. His explanation was that the "care" was outside of his office, and he'd forgotten to tell his bookkeeper. Although she said she'd changed jobs and health insurance companies in the interim, he would not cancel the bill. She decided to make him wait for payment—until dunned by a collection agency. She paid, but changed doctors.

Ways to Reduce Medical Costs

More than half of the almost $100 billion paid annually for health care in the United States goes to hospitals, where 32 million people are attended each year. Yet only 10 to 20 percent of all health care is delivered in hospitals, and only $1 out of every $6 paid to a hospital is used for patient care.

It is estimated that 30 percent of the patients in hospitals have no need to be there. Health insurance companies once required patients to be hospitalized in order to receive benefits. Many a physician developed the habit of putting moderately sick patients into hospitals so expenses would be paid by the insurance company. If the doctor owned a share of the hospital or received a fee for each admission, he was willing. Now health insurance companies are offering many types of policies to cover care that does not require hospitalization. These policies save money for insurance companies—and for you.

The overuse of hospital beds is receiving attention, as is the distribution of hospitals. Rural areas generally lack ample facilities and doctors. Populous areas often have overcrowding in some hospitals and too many empty beds in other hospitals within the same city.

Many hospitals are trying to cooperate by increasing outpatient and ambulatory care and emergency facilities, by revamping procedures, by sharing expensive new equipment with other hospitals in the vicinity, and by other innovations.

If you are scheduled for elective (nonemergency) surgery, you can take preadmission tests as an outpatient, going home instead of occupying a hospital bed between tests and while tests are being analyzed. You need not be admitted to the hospital for "preop" preparation until the afternoon before major surgery is scheduled.

Minor surgery is often performed in the morning. You may rest for a while, then go home or to a hotel without having to spend one night in a hospital. This can cut your bill by one third.

Progressive-care plans in some hospitals promote patients as they improve. Patients move from intensive or coronary care units with constant monitoring and five hours a day of nursing attention . . . to a regular room . . . to a minimum care unit where patients bathe and dress themselves, eat in a dining room, and go to therapy departments for appointments.

Patients hospitalized for illness or surgery are now released earlier than used to be customary. Barring complications, a five-day stay for major abdominal surgery is not unusual. Patients are not permitted to lie in bed all day, weakening their muscles. As necessary, doctors transfer them to nursing homes, arrange for home nursing services, or explain recuperative home care to patients and their families.

Alternatives to hospitals for patients who do not need hospital beds or costly equipment for tests and therapy are the growing number of medical centers in neighborhoods or small towns. Mainly group-practice clinics, these centers often have an emergency room, examining rooms, a testing laboratory, and one or more surgical suites for minor surgery on outpatients.

Part of the rising cost for medical care is due to unnecessary duplication of tests. When you have occasion to see another doctor soon after tests were made, this records book will show test results or indicate where X rays and complex data are stored. However, if you take certain medications for a long time, blood tests are essential at regular intervals to measure the levels of the drug in your blood to show whether a change in dosage is needed. Blood tests can also indicate whether the medicine may be damaging the liver or another part of the body.

Often a new doctor routinely orders "workups"—every diagnostic test he or she thinks might apply or simply to have proof of a patient's condition when first consulted. Show him your records and ask why more tests are necessary. He may present sound reasons to explain how new tests will benefit you—or be angry that you dare question his orders. In the latter event, consider whether you want this person as your new doctor. One out of three X rays (costing $3 billion a year) are made for the doctor's protection, exposing patients to needless radiation hazards.

Before arrangements are made for extensive treatment, frankly discuss the costs. You may have to talk with the nurse or secretary, who may relay questions and answers, for many doctors do not wish to appear undignified by speaking of money.

Your bills could mount up to high figures for special diagnostic tests or medication, fees for surgery or consultations or a series of office visits, a long hospital stay, a private room, rehabilitation therapy, or whatever is applicable to your illness. If costs are more than you can afford, even on an extended payment basis, don't be embarrassed to say so. Perhaps there are alternatives. Examples: Automated multiphasic testing costs less than individual tests as a hospital inpatient or outpatient. Generic drugs, when available in the medication needed, cost less than brand-name ones. If your doctor is going to give you a prescription for penicillin tablets or capsules, for instance, don't hesitate to ask him to write the generic "penicillin" instead of a brand name.

Keep your appointments with doctors or you may be charged as a "no-show," especially by dentists and other specialists who work on schedules that allocate a specific amount of time per patient. To

24

avoid waiting in a physician's office when you are very busy, you might phone to find out whether the physician is on schedule and can see you at the appointed time.

Get to know your body and think clearly about any health problem. Although doctors belittle self-diagnosis, you must know the importance of symptoms because you are the one who decides when you need professional care, and your physician relies, to some extent, on what you relate.

Some people, especially men, practice fortitude and will silently endure pain for a long time. They are denying disease. They think it is a sign of weakness to admit they don't feel well and need medical help. When members of their families suggest they see a doctor, they are often too obstinate to do so. Trying to ignore pain, a major symptom of most diseases, or the painless symptoms of other diseases may be fatal. Also, individuals who have some natural tolerance for pain need to become aware of when their pain rises to a level that requires medical attention.

Physicians often classify patients as "the well, the worried well, the early sick, and the sick." When you are among the sick or early sick or have had an accident, see your doctor promptly. However, some physicians say half of the office visits are unnecessary; others note that general practitioners spend from 70 to 85 percent of their time on "the well or worried well." In these cases there is no discoverable organic disease. The basic problem is likely to be emotional—but that problem may cause physical symptoms and, eventually, disorders. One way a psychosomatic illness can develop is when you hear about a disease that intrigues the mind into suggesting that the body duplicate the symptoms. If you continually think about getting a disorder, your subconscious may try to make it a fact.

"You are not as sick as you think" is the sign on one doctor's wall. Why not discard the words "suffer" and "victim of a disease" from your vocabulary?

Patients take up doctors' time because they want attention, sympathy, or a feeling of importance by having extra "special" tests. They do a disservice to themselves and doctors. With the shortage of physicians, some doctors work from 60 to 100 hours a week and don't have time to give more than a prescription for temporary euphoria— the overused tranquilizer. Really sick people await their care.

Let your own good common sense and knowledge of health guide you on when to see a physician. Try additional interests to dispel self-concern and baseless anxiety about severe illness. After all, when you read about 55,000 fatalities in vehicular accidents the previous year, that doesn't stop you from entering an automobile. You look at it this way: 212,945,000 Americans rode safely. So fasten your seat belt, drive carefully, and enjoy the ride. Take precautions against illness, too, but enjoy living.

Checkpoints to Guard Your Health

Always wear an identification (ID) bracelet or neck tag if you have a health problem that may not be apparent. It will call attention to your immediate need for proper medical care when you cannot communicate because you are deaf, blind, unconscious, confused, delirious, hysterical, in a coma or state of shock.

ID bracelets or neck tags should be worn by the one out of five persons who has a "hidden" medical problem. Heart conditions, severe allergies, diabetes, and epilepsy are the most usual of the 200 reasons. Significant allergies could include many drugs commonly used in emergencies, such as penicillin, sulfa, morphine, codeine, and tetanus serum.

Other medical problems appropriate to an ID tag include asthma, glaucoma, chorea (St. Vitus's dance and other involuntary motions), hemophilia (tendency to bleed profusely even from a small cut). Also to be noted are whether a person has an implanted pacemaker, has had a tracheostomy and is a neck breather, has a rare blood type, wears contact lenses that could cause scarring of the cornea after 36 hours, is allergic to feather pillows or to insect stings and has not been desensitized, is deaf or mentally retarded, is a scuba diver, is taking anticoagulants, cortisone, heart drugs, thyroid, or other medications. If the person does not speak English, the ID should show what language(s) are understood. It is also a good idea to wear an ID noting pregnancy during the early months, especially if a woman has a history of eclampsia, miscarriages, or other complication.

Consult your physician to find out whether you should wear emergency ID and what conditions should be cited. Record all circumstances that must be known promptly on the "Emergency?" pages of this book so anyone in your family can give them quickly by phone. Carry the book with you when you travel.

An ID bracelet is more obvious than a neck tag to someone who comes to see what's wrong. An ID neck tag will be seen when a collar or other clothing is loosened if fainting seems to be the problem at first. Jewelry stores sell suitable bracelets and neck tags and will handle the engraving, or you can obtain them from sources described later in this section.

A wallet card, giving full information, should also be carried. The cards supplied with wallets usually do not allow sufficient space. You can type or print your own card and fold it to fit in your wallet. You can buy a plastic ID wallet card that includes some of your medical records on microfilm, but they cannot be read without a high-powered magnifying instrument.

Two nonprofit organizations which will supply emergency protection services for small, tax-deductible sums are Medic Alert and Medi-Check. Both use the quickly identified medical symbol of a snake on a rod and the three cross bars denoting emergency. Although the purpose of both organizations is the same, the methods employed and materials supplied are different. To assure accuracy in your identification, write one of the organizations for a form.

Medi-Check International Foundation, 2640 Golf Road, Glenview, Ill. 60025, suggests a minimum donation of $2.50 for a bracelet and $2 for either a neck tag or wallet card. Made of stainless steel, the metal recommended for diabetics and least likely to cause an allergy, the bracelet or neck tag can be engraved with eight lines of copy. An example: Your name, street address, city and state, area code and phone number on four lines; "allergic to penicillin" on two lines, and your doctor's name and phone number on two lines. The wallet card in durable aluminum will contain your name, address, and phone number in four lines on the front and can carry eight longer lines giving whatever information you wish on the back.

Medic Alert Foundation International, Turlock, Calif. 95380, offers a lifetime membership. The fee is based on the metal used for the bracelet or necklace. It is $7 for stainless steel, $12 for sterling silver, or $28 for 10K gold. The reverse side is engraved with the Medic Alert emergency phone number, the member's ID number, and the "hidden" medical problem or problems. Four fourteen-character lines can be engraved. The first line is included in the fee; additional lines are 75¢ each. A dated cardboard wallet card containing additional medical and personal information is supplied annually or whenever changes require a new card.

Medic Alert maintains an emergency answering system which can give, through the retrieval of computerized data, all emergency information on a member to medical personnel who call collect to the phone number on the bracelet or necklace and wallet card.

The organization figures the average number of "hidden" medical problems per member is 2.3. In a recent twelve-month period, over 2,000 members reported the system helped save their lives.

Have a complete physical checkup regularly. How often? How complete? It depends upon your age, occupation, individual health records, and family health history. After the pediatric stage, when children's diseases are treated, and after puberty, when acne problems and endocrine changes may need attention, a healthy twenty-year-old person with a moderate lifestyle should have a really complete examination to record his normal health, then have checkups as needed until age forty.

Starting around forty, annual checkups are recommended. Yet a survey of high-income men over this age showed a third had checkups every year, a third every three to five years, and the remaining third only when hospitalized—too late for preventive medicine. The purpose of a checkup is to catch a disorder before it gets a real start.

By age sixty-five, checkups should be scheduled for every six months or more frequently when required by a chronic condition. Regular examinations are suggested, although the elderly average only 1.3 acute illnesses a year, about half the rate for the entire population. Accidents are usually due to decreased vision, hearing, and mobility.

While Medicare covers much of the cost for illnesses, it can do little to screen for developing conditions. Some hospitals are starting to fill this need by offering a series of low-cost examinations after peak periods for staff and facilities. The schedule one month may be for blood tests, another month for electrocardiograms, and so on. If this service is not available in your community, find out whether there is an automated multiphasic testing center. Multiple tests are given in an assembly-line system, but this service requires little time and money. In either method, test results are sent to the patient's own physician.

Written reports on laboratory tests are sufficient for your physician, but ask that X-ray films and any electrodiagnoses recorded on sensitized or graph-type paper be sent to your own physician for study before being filed at the hospital or clinic. Although X-ray films of fractures and organs are examined carefully by orthopedic and other surgeons, chest X rays are rarely seen by general physicians.

On many diagnostic tests, doctors usually receive a nonspecific word report: "Not enough evidence to justify further studies" or "No significant abnormalities." Such a report was sent to one man's doctor after the man had a chest X ray. Five months later two of the three lobes of his right lung were found malignant and removed.

Another man who had had routine chest X rays for years did not know he had an enlarged heart until his physician saw his X ray in the hospital to which he was sent in an ambulance after a heart attack. A smoker with a chronic cough relied on annual chest X rays to check on her lungs. She did not know she had osteoporosis and a lateral curvature of the spine until the doctor at a new testing clinic pointed them out on her chest X ray.

The U.S. Comptroller General's Report to Congress entitled "Public Hazards from Unsatisfactory Medical Diagnostic Products," dated April 30, 1975, notes: "Today more than ever, doctors are relying on laboratory tests to help diagnose, treat, or control medical conditions and diseases. An inaccurate diagnosis may result in injury to an individual's health; death; or, at a minimum, needless medical expense. Unreliable diagnostic products contribute to inaccurate laboratory test results."

The Center for Disease Control of the Department of Health, Education, and Welfare evaluated *in vitro* diagnostic products. These are chemical or biological substances, kits, or instruments used to examine a specimen for the presence or absence of a disease or condition. The Report to Congress states: "Center officials estimate that 25 percent (about 750 million) of all diagnostic test results are unreliable and that erroneous diagnostic tests result in, among other things, unnecessary medical treatment, withholding necessary medical treatment, and lost income, costing the U.S. economy $25 billion annually."

The Food and Drug Administration's regulations provide for voluntary registration of manufacturers and for the establishment of performance and labeling standards. The FDA's regulatory activities have been declared ineffective. Concerned about rates of error, 14,000 independent and hospital laboratories are making an effort to develop standard references for chemical analyses and to calibrate laboratory instruments uniformly. Human errors, such as mislabeling of body serums, also occur. If you have doubts about any test result, tell your doctor you would like the test repeated.

Especially for your primary physician or dentist, choose wisely. On the recommendation of a friend in the city to which he had moved, a man had a thorough physical examination, electrocardiogram, and laboratory and other tests in the doctor's offices to establish his records while healthy. A year later he became ill but could find no trace of the physician or his records.

A woman went to her dentist every six months for eight years. During the last three years she told him on every visit that her gums bled when she brushed her teeth and asked whether she had gingivitis or periodontitis. He assured her she did not. A month after a regular checkup, a section of a tooth broke off, and she phoned for an appointment. The man had retired and turned over his records to another dentist. The new dentist asked, "When are you going to have your periodontal disease treated?" On two-year-old X rays, he pointed out how obvious the disease was. Phoning the retired dentist at his home, she was told the periodontitis must have developed very quickly. Finally, the dentist admitted he had been going blind.

The halos of some doctors are slipping. It has been acknowledged that 5 percent are drug addicts, alcoholics, or have serious mental disorders. States vary in licensing standards, but, once licensed, doctors are not reexamined for fitness to practice.

A comparison: Commercial airline pilots must have complete physical examinations by a Federal Aviation Administration flight surgeon twice a year. Some airlines require a third examination. The pilots' health is checked after any illness. They are watched and tested to find out whether they are adopting any bad habits. Their flying ability is examined every six months and spot-checked between tests. They are constantly retrained, sometimes using computer-assisted simulators of flight conditions, to reveal their split-second reactions. The most experienced pilots start from scratch to learn all about a different type of plane before they are permitted to fly it.

Rarely does a doctor devote the recommended hour to taking a patient's health history. Yet, as one physician commented, "Doctors who don't have a patient's history take a shortcut to a guess diagnosis." Be sure *your* doctors know your health history by gathering previous facts, adding current and future data, and taking your health records book with you on every visit to any doctor.

Although doctors may have honest differences of opinion on therapy, the diagnosis must be accurate. Yet sometimes diseases are difficult to diagnose at first. Clues may be well hidden. Symptoms (subjective) described by the patient or observed by the doctor, and signs (objective) found by the doctor during his examination and in tests, may add up to syndromes that could indicate any of several diseases.

Finding what seems to be an unusual disease can sometimes be as exciting for a doctor as turning up a rare potsherd is to an archeologist. But do you want to be tagged with a rare disease and be treated for a condition that may not exist? If you have any doubt about a diagnosis and your doctor does not arrange a consultation, you may wish to consult another doctor to avoid possible misdiagnosis or overdiagnosis, mistreatment or overtreatment, or overuse of the scalpel.

Whether or not you tell your first doctor you are consulting another, he should not object to peer review. Take all health records with you when you visit the doctor you are consulting. If this doctor makes the same diagnosis and suggests the same therapy as your regular doctor did, you may feel more assured.

Although there is a shortage of general physicians, currently there is an oversupply of surgeons. It has been estimated that up to one quarter of the multimillion operations performed each year are unnecessary. Board-certified specialists at a leading medical college, examining 1,356 patients recommended for surgery, found that 24 percent of all operations was not needed; 40 percent of the recommended orthopedic (joints and spine) surgery was not necessary.

Per 100,000 members of the population, the number of operations is directly related to the number of surgeons and hospitals in various regions of the United States. The types of operations also vary with geography. Why should there be more operations on eyes, ears, nose, throat, and breasts in the Midwest than in the other regions? Why is surgery on the spine and heart valves highest in the West?

Why be rushed into elective (nonemergency) surgery? Be cautious if a surgeon says your particular condition has no priority in obtaining a hospital bed if the condition should suddenly become an emergency. With this unnerving prospect—and unaware that there are empty hospital beds—many people consent to surgery on tonsils, adenoids, appendices, uteri, gall bladders, and other "removable parts," without checking first with other surgeons and without asking questions about the risks involved or alternative therapy. Many surgeons and patients think that literally cutting out a problem will solve it. Surgery is not always that definitive.

Many hospitals have review committees that check on samples of tissue removed during surgery and the pathology reports to ascertain whether a particular surgeon makes too many errors in diagnoses. This peer review is *after operations,* too late for the patients who may have had needless surgery. Anesthesia and surgery are traumas (shocks; severe wounds) to any body.

Groups with prepaid medical plans (see Health Maintenance Organizations in this book), being more interested in disease prevention, average one surgeon per 12,471 people. For the general public there is one surgeon per 7,573 people.

Drug Interactions

Before prescribing a medicine, a doctor must know what the patient is currently taking under other doctors' orders or if alcohol or diet pills are being used. Many drugs increase, decrease, or otherwise change the action of many other drugs, though each may accomplish its purpose when taken alone.

To avoid drug interactions, some pharmacists are starting patient record files. If a pharmacist takes time to check these files and detects a possible interaction, he phones the doctor, and you must get a new prescription. Do you have all of yours filled at the same place?

In most of Europe and in the Americas, except the United States, laws require that pharmaceutical labels include brand and generic names, indications (what the medication is for), ingredients, possible side effects, full dosage range, and expiration date if there is one. Because drugs are prepackaged by the manufacturers in the most frequently prescribed units, patients receive all these helpful facts.

In the United States, knowledge is often deliberately withheld from patients on what drugs they are taking, the therapeutic purposes, and the possible side effects. Without lists of ingredients, patients cannot help in detecting what specific ones in several compounds may cause their adverse reactions.

Respect those powerful little pills and capsules. They can be beneficial or harmful. It is estimated that between 18 and 20 percent of all patients have adverse drug reactions in hospitals and 4 to 6 percent of all hospital admissions are due to adverse drug reactions. One hospital day in seven is spent in the care of drug toxicity, at the annual cost of $3 billion. The U.S. Public Health Service estimates that 1,300,000 "therapeutic misadventures" occur each year.

Those figures pertain to legally prescribed drugs. Here are examples of the deadliness of street-sold drugs: At the University of Southern California Medical School it was found that pep pills (amphetamines) blocked small arteries, causing strokes and deaths among young users. In Chicago during 1974, 456 people died from illegal drugs.

You may have heard the word "placebo" (pronounced "plah-see'-boe"). Placebos are harmless, do-nothing pills made of inert matter or distilled-water injections. Occasionally doctors give placebos to patients who demand something for a slight illness or more medication than is safe. Placebos often have a psychological effect and can help relieve pain or permit sleep.

Placebos are mainly used for the "control group" when a new

drug is being tested. Research doctors and persons taking placebos or the actual medication do not know which is which because they are made to look alike. This is done to assure accuracy in appraising the effects of the medicine. The testing of some new drugs takes around five years. Proof of efficacy is needed by the pharmaceutical manufacturer to obtain Food and Drug Administration approval to market the drug.

This is one reason for the time lapse between news articles on a medical discovery and the availability of the drug or technique. Patients often rush to their doctors with newspaper clippings in their hands, wanting the foretold benefits right away. They do not realize how much time it takes, after research and initial testing on animals or a limited number of human volunteers, to prove the value of a new drug and to show it does not have harmful effects on most people.

Applied science, government agencies, and the medical profession "make haste slowly." Most doctors hesitate to use something new, something their colleagues are not already using, lest they be considered nonconformists. Detail men (pharmaceutical manufacturers' representatives who call on doctors) say doctors are interested in the details of new discoveries but slow to try them. They also complain it is difficult to switch a doctor from a drug he or she customarily prescribes because the doctor knows its effects.

General inertia is partly to blame for the slow acceptance of a new medication. It often takes a crisis or pressure from the public to speed up matters. For instance, penicillin was first made in 1928, but not until World War II did it gain wide acceptance. Now it is the antibiotic of choice by most doctors—unless they know a patient is allergic to it.

The benefits of keeping your own records are virtually endless. Doctors who do not have adequate files on you can be alerted to possible problems. Examples: A gynecologist could note that a patient's blood pressure has not been checked for a long time. A dentist could see a patient is taking an anticoagulant and check with the physician or be extra cautious in an extraction. An anesthetist or anesthesiologist must know what drugs you have been taking, especially barbiturates or any CNS (central nervous system) depressants.

Put Facts at Your Fingertips

Do you know the names and locations of organs, bones, and teeth so you can tell the doctor on the phone where you hurt? Check the illustrations in this book.

Do you know where your X rays are stored?

Did you have X-ray treatments between the late 1930s and early 1950s for acne or on tonsils, adenoids, thymus, or lymph glands? If so, respond to the pleas of hospitals searching for former patients to whom they gave radiation treatments, acceptable at that time, but later found capable of producing thyroid tumors.

Have you ever looked in vain for a copy of your lens prescription to take along in case you break or lose eyeglasses on a trip?

When schools and camps request them, can you find records of childhood diseases and immunizations for each of your children?

When you are exposed to a childhood disease more severe in adults, do you know whether you are immune because you've had it?

For an insurance application, can you remember quickly what surgery you had and when?

If you feel overly anxious about any disease you read about that might be hereditary, do you know whether any of your forebears had it?

Whatever your age, be a detective and recorder—now. At some time your life could be saved or its quality improved because of significant facts in this registry. Accurately fill in the facts you know. If you prefer to omit your age or other pertinent data, be sure to *tell* each doctor. Find out all you can from your relatives about your health heritage, childhood diseases, and immunizations. Start now and continue recording facts as you obtain them.

Get in touch with previous doctors. Their files may be hiding data vital to your present and future health care. If they decline to release information directly to you, have it sent to your present primary physician. He can direct his aide or nurse to enter data or give them to you for this book. Ask all of your present doctors to make relevant entries at the times you see them. If they are of the new breed, they realize that lack of communication can be more devastating in health care than in almost any other area.

Your personal health biography will be as useful as you and your doctors make it. It's up to you to fill in most of the blank spaces. But it's your health, isn't it?

This Is I

Name at birth _____

If name changed through marriage or court approval:

_____

date   name changed to

_____

date   name changed to

_____

date   name changed to

                                                         A.M.

Birth date _____ P.M.

       year   month   date   hour

Birth place _____

             name of hospital; home; other

Attending physician _____

If any problems at birth _____

Birth recorded at _____

(name of place) Department of Public Health; county courthouse; other

_____

           state   date

Birth recorded by _____

            name of hospital; doctor; parent; other

Position in family (e.g., 2nd of 3 children) _____

Age of parents at birth: Mother _____ . **Father** _____ .

Mother _____

        given name   maiden name   married name

Father _____

        given name   middle name   surname

Maybe in My Genes

Some descendants—not all—may inherit a tendency toward a family weakness. If your doctor knows of a disorder in your blood line, he examines you thoroughly for it. If he assures you that you have no signs of the condition, relax. Significant chromosomal defects or chemical deficiencies in babies (which happens 1 time out of every 200) can now be detected before birth and in some cases treated.

Note relationship (mother, uncle, grandparent, other)

Allergies _____

Arthritis _____

Bronchial asthma _____

Cancer _____

Color-blindness _____

Cystic fibrosis _____

Diabetes _____

Glaucoma _____

Gout _____

Hemophilia _____

High blood pressure _____

Migraine headaches _____

Pernicious anemia _____

Severe drug reactions (name drugs) _____

_____

_____

Sickle-cell anemia _____

Skin disorders: psoriasis, ichthyosis, atopic dermatitis _____

Other _____

_____

Lifetimes in My Family Tree

If your ancestors fell out at a ripe old age, you may expect a long life, too. But don't give up if they didn't reach ninety. Medical advancements and an individual's interest in health care can extend life. Show the longevity of recent parentage below. If this is a youngster's health record, and all are now living, leave blank except for parents' heights and weights.

	Age at death	Cause of death
Maternal grandfather (mother's father)	_____	_____
Maternal grandmother (mother's mother)	_____	_____
Paternal grandfather (father's father)	_____	_____
Paternal grandmother (father's mother)	_____	_____
Father	_____	_____
Mother	_____	_____
Brother	_____	_____
Brother	_____	_____
Sister	_____	_____
Sister	_____	_____

Heights of mother _____; **father** _____

Average weights of mother _____; **father** _____

How I Grew—Upward and Outward

Take height in bare feet. Weigh yourself in the morning, after voiding, before breakfast. One formula to show *average* gains for children: At age two, a girl has reached 52 percent of her adult height, a boy 48.5 percent; at age twelve, a girl is 77.6 percent of her adult height, a boy 84 percent of his. A baby who gains around 12 pounds (5.5 kilograms) in the first six months after birth may be a "fatty" unless put on a diet, but have a doctor examine the baby.

Age	Height	Weight	Age	Height	Weight

Infectious Diseases I Have Had

Many infectious diseases build up immunity. Some can attack again. Others leave long-lasting disturbances in the body. If you had any of these diseases, mark an X or fill in the year.

Acute influenza _____	**Relapsing fever** _____
Amebiasis _____	**Rheumatic fever** _____
Chicken pox _____	**Rickets** _____
Cholera _____	**Scarlet fever** _____
Diphtheria _____	**Smallpox** _____
Encephalitis _____	**Spirochetal jaundice** _____
Enterovirus disease _____	**Staph infection** _____
German measles _____	**Strep infection** _____
Infectious chorea _____	**Systemic fungus** _____
Infectious hepatitis _____	**Tetanus** _____
Malaria _____	**Trichiniasis** _____
Measles _____	**Tuberculosis** _____
Meningitis _____	**Typhoid** _____
Mononucleosis _____	**Typhus** _____
Mumps _____	**Venereal disease** _____
Paratyphoid _____	**Virus pneumonia** _____
Plague _____	**Whooping cough** _____
Polio _____	**Yellow fever** _____

Others _____

Immunizations for the prevention of communicable diseases are also called shots, inoculations, or vaccinations. Polio immunizations may be Sabin oral vaccine or Salk injected vaccine. Sometimes shots are combined—e.g., DTP is diphtheria, tetanus, and pertussis (whooping cough). When you are immunized against an allergy or influenza, be specific. Record each time a shot is given, whether it's a booster or one of a series. For example, DTP and typhoid require three injections; polio needs two oral doses. List your immunizations on the next page.

Immunizations Record

Date	Immunization	Physician giving

In Hospital for Illness or Accident

Reason _____ _____

Dates _____ _____

Doctor _____ _____

Hospital _____ _____

City _____ _____

Reason _____ _____

Dates _____ _____

Doctor _____ _____

Hospital _____ _____

City _____ _____

Reason _____ _____

Dates _____ _____

Doctor _____ _____

Hospital _____ _____

City _____ _____

Reason _____ _____

Dates _____ _____

Doctor _____ _____

Hospital _____ _____

City _____ _____

Reason _____ _____

Dates _____ _____

Doctor _____ _____

Hospital _____ _____

City _____ _____

Surgery Performed on Me

Surgery _____   _____

Date _____   _____

Surgeon _____   _____

Hospital _____   _____

City _____   _____

Surgery _____   _____

Date _____   _____

Surgeon _____   _____

Hospital _____   _____

City _____   _____

Surgery _____   _____

Date _____   _____

Surgeon _____   _____

Hospital _____   _____

City _____   _____

Surgery _____   _____

Date _____   _____

Surgeon _____   _____

Hospital _____   _____

City _____   _____

Surgery _____   _____

Date _____   _____

Surgeon _____   _____

Hospital _____   _____

City _____   _____

Multiple diagnostic tests, with information stored in computers, are given by some hospitals, clinics, physician groups, and public health services. The systems are designated as AMHT (automated multiphasic health testing), MHS (multiple health screening), or some similar name. The purpose is to give well or nearly well people a comprehensive examination that may detect a hidden ailment.

Screening tests save time for physicians who are too busy diagnosing and treating diseases to check for possible oncoming disorders, and they give specialists information on the general health of their patients. The tests make people more health-conscious and could prevent serious illness by showing possible problems for doctors to check on more thoroughly. When required, treatment can start in the earliest stages of a disorder.

A simplified summary of the testing: At a computer console, you push buttons to answer questions on your family and personal health and to assess your own state of health. Most examinees use 150 to 200 questions, though the computers can ask over 350. Doctors, technicians, and electronic devices make these physical tests:

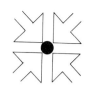

Multiple Screening Tests

1. Blood pressure and pulse rate are taken.
2. An electocardiogram is made to show the heart's activity.
3. An X ray of the chest reveals the condition of lungs, heart size, and density of bones in the rib cage.
4. Sight is checked for acuity in each eye and in both eyes, farsightedness or nearsightedness, vertical and lateral vision, ocular tension, color and depth perception. Eyes are not tested for lenses.
5. Hearing loss for each ear and both ears is tested by a precision audiometer. Wearing earphones, you press a device to record how well you hear sound frequencies in low, middle, and high ranges.
6. Lung capacity is measured in terms of forced and timed vital capacities as you blow into a spirometer.
7. Anthropometric measurements are taken for height, weight, and skinfold thickness.
8. Laboratory tests are made on specimens of blood, urine, and feces. Blood is drawn there; the others are brought in by the examinee, who receives instructions prior to testing.
9. Doctors give general physical and proctoscopic examinations. Women have a gynecology examination and a Papanicolaou test (the so-called "Pap smear" which enables the early detection of uterine cancer).

10. Breast thermography for women (and some men) is now included in regular tests by many centers. If the doctors determine a woman (or a man) should have X-ray mammography, this is arranged at an additional fee for the same or another day.

Some clinics substitute glucose tolerance, oral health, or other tests for a few of the tests mentioned here.

Testing takes an examinee around three hours. If you wish, you may return two weeks later for an interpretation of test results by a clinic doctor at no extra charge. All information is stored in the computer, and print-outs are sent only to the doctor or doctors you authorize to receive the data. Multiple-screening is a fast, economical way to take many diagnostic tests; however, your doctors may want additional or confirmatory tests.

You will certainly want more tests if the screening clinic reports "emphysema," for instance, on the basis of only two exhalations into the spirometer and chest X rays interpreted by someone who is not a specialist. One examinee borrowed the X rays, had pulmonary screening tests as a hospital outpatient, and saw a pulmonary disease specialist. He said the patient had mild bronchitis but there was no sign of emphysema.

Despite occasional misinterpretations by testing center personnel, rectifiable by one's own physician, multiple screening programs are effective. They offer people their only opportunity for regular checkups or give more tests than the usual checkups—and they do so in less time and at lower cost than any other method. Screening tests can detect clues to developing ailments, alerting patients and their physicians. Doctors often obtain better patient histories than in interviews because people respond more frankly to questions on the computer, and it gives them time to think or revise first answers.

The computer records will not substitute for those in this book. Questions on medical history asked at the computer console are not sufficiently precise to apply to each individual. Medicines are grouped. Times of health problems are often limited to "over three years ago." Some clinics retain records for only five years or transfer them to microfilm. To have print-outs made for another doctor at a later date, if data are still available, you must first sign a release and pay an additional fee to the testing center. You can avoid delay and extra cost by copying the important data in your own record book.

If you have had multiphasic tests, fill in the form on the next page. Record facts from those tests and additional diagnostic tests on the ensuing pages. Otherwise skip directly to the next sections.

Multiple Screening Tests

It is recommended tests be repeated every twelve to eighteen months. Dates tests were made:

_____ _____ _____ _____ _____ _____

_____ _____ _____ _____ _____ _____

_____ _____ _____ _____ _____ _____

_____ _____ _____ _____ _____ _____

_____ _____ _____ _____ _____ _____

Hospital or clinic where tests were made and data are stored:

Name _____

Address, City, State _____

When you move and use other health screening services:

Name _____

Address, City, State _____

Name _____

Address, City, State _____

Doctors who have computerized print-outs on screening tests:

Doctor _____   _____

Address _____   _____

City, State _____   _____

Phone _____   _____

Doctor _____   _____

Address _____   _____

City, State _____   _____

Phone _____   _____

Of the 23 to 24 million Americans who have high blood pressure (hypertension), only half know they have it and only one tenth have it under control. High blood pressure is a major cause of deaths from heart diseases (about 750,000) and strokes (over 200,000) annually, according to Vital Statistics of the United States. Hypertension is said by some sources to be the primary cause of another 60,000 deaths a year. It contributes to deaths from kidney and other diseases. Directly or indirectly, high blood pressure accounts for over half the mortality rate in the United States.

These statistics are given only to emphasize the importance of having your blood pressure checked, to "perform a death-defying act," as the American Heart Association advises.

Your doctor has at his or her command a large variety of drugs to lower blood pressure. In some cases the doctor can find out, before prescribing, what is causing the elevation and select a specific medication with a specific action. Sometimes the reason for hypertension is not apparent or there may be several factors. If you have any side effects from the drug your doctor prescribed, don't just stop taking it. Phone the doctor immediately. He or she can adjust the dosage or change to another medicine that may be more appropriate for you.

Having blood pressure checked frequently and bringing it under control if it is high is your best insurance for a healthier, longer life. In fact, insurance companies use blood pressure as a criterion for life expectancies. If it is inconvenient for you to go to your physician's office as often as seems necessary or if your blood pressure goes up in anxious anticipation, your doctor may train someone in your family to take your blood pressure on a home unit.

Blood pressure is the force exerted by flowing blood against the walls of arteries. It is measured with a sphygmomanometer, better known as the B.P. cuff, though the device also has an air bulb pump, valve, and pressure gauge. A stethoscope is needed.

The person operating the sphygmomanometer winds the cloth cuff with its hollow pocket for air around your upper arm and pumps in air by contracting the bulb until the expanded cuff temporarily stops the flow of blood. When the examiner hears this through the stethoscope, he releases air pressure until the heartbeat can be heard again. The reading at this point is the higher (systolic) measurement—the chambers of the heart are emptying themselves of blood. Releasing more air from the cuff, he hears the beat get louder, then fade. When the sound disappears, the heart is relaxing. This is the lower (diastolic) reading—the chambers are refilling with blood.

Blood pressure varies with sex and age. Even infants can have high blood pressure. In the same person blood pressure has many temporary fluctuations—decreasing during sleep or relaxation, increasing with physical exertion, excitement, anger, etc. When blood pressure is continuously high, a person has hypertension. Low blood pressure is called hypotension. Normal pressure ranges are around 90 to 140 for systolic (the first number obtained in a reading) and 60 to 90 for diastolic (the second number). Diastolic pressure above 90 is the more serious if it is consistently high. A chronological sequence of readings is very informative.

Blood Pressure Readings

Date	Pressures	Date	Pressures	Date	Pressures
_____	___/___	_____	___/___	_____	___/___
_____	___/___	_____	___/___	_____	___/___
_____	___/___	_____	___/___	_____	___/___
_____	___/___	_____	___/___	_____	___/___
_____	___/___	_____	___/___	_____	___/___
_____	___/___	_____	___/___	_____	___/___
_____	___/___	_____	___/___	_____	___/___
_____	___/___	_____	___/___	_____	___/___
_____	___/___	_____	___/___	_____	___/___
_____	___/___	_____	___/___	_____	___/___
_____	___/___	_____	___/___	_____	___/___
_____	___/___	_____	___/___	_____	___/___
_____	___/___	_____	___/___	_____	___/___
_____	___/___	_____	___/___	_____	___/___
_____	___/___	_____	___/___	_____	___/___
_____	___/___	_____	___/___	_____	___/___
_____	___/___	_____	___/___	_____	___/___
_____	___/___	_____	___/___	_____	___/___

Enter your basic blood type when you know for sure:

Blood group____. (O, A, B, or AB)

About 85 percent of humans have the Rh factor. It is important to know whether one has Rh positive or Rh negative blood for blood transfusions and during pregnancies when mother and fetus have different factors. Rh positive is the most common. Blood can also have other factors, such as M, N, and P. Wear an ID bracelet or neck tag if you have a rare blood type and check here:

Rh negative____. M____. N____. P____. Other____.

Whatever your blood type, note it in the "Emergency?" section.

Because blood discloses many facts about how your body is functioning and whether the dosage of a medicine is right for you, your doctor orders blood analyses. The frequency depends upon what is being checked. Although specific tests can be made, these two fairly comprehensive tests are the most usual:

1. *CBC (complete blood count):* It gives the number or percentage and types of red and white blood corpuscles and of platelets. These are the solid components of blood.
2. *Survey-12:* Many laboratories in hospitals or clinics have two analyzers to enable them to make up to twenty-four tests at the same time. These measure proteins, glucose, cholesterol, uric acid, sodium, calcium, phosphate, other chemicals in the blood.

Normally, a cubic millimeter of blood has 4 to 5 million red blood cells in women, 4.5 to 5.5 million in men, and 5,000 to 10,000 white blood cells. If the count of white blood cells is higher, it shows they have multiplied to fight an infection somewhere in the body. The platelet count is from 200,000 to 800,000 per cubic millimeter.

Normal ranges per 100 milliliters for other analyses which may interest you are: Glucose (sugar) 80 to 120 milligrams, uric acid 3 to 5 milligrams, and cholesterol 150 to 250 milligrams. Variations from some norms are allowed for age, sex, and weight.

The only test findings that need be recorded are those significant to a disorder for which you are being treated—e.g., diabetes (high glucose level), hypoglycemia (low glucose level), gout (uric acid in blood), anemia, liver disorders, blood levels high in cholesterol and triglycerides (blood fats), acidosis, alkalosis, or others. Your sequential records make it easier for your family doctor to check and could be important to various specialists you visit. Because diet, as well as medicine, is part of the treatment for these disorders, you have considerable control and will want to watch the progress being made.

48

Blood Analyses

Date	Test for	Count or %
————	————————————————————	————
————	————————————————————	————
————	————————————————————	————
————	————————————————————	————
————	————————————————————	————
————	————————————————————	————
————	————————————————————	————
————	————————————————————	————
————	————————————————————	————
————	————————————————————	————
————	————————————————————	————
————	————————————————————	————
————	————————————————————	————
————	————————————————————	————
————	————————————————————	————
————	————————————————————	————
————	————————————————————	————
————	————————————————————	————
————	————————————————————	————
————	————————————————————	————
————	————————————————————	————
————	————————————————————	————
————	————————————————————	————
————	————————————————————	————

X Rays, Fluoroscopes, Isotopes

When a physicist named Roentgen discovered short light waves in 1895, he called them X rays because of their unknown nature. Since then, knowledge has expanded vastly, but all is not yet known about the beneficial uses, the mutation or destruction of tissues from over-exposure, or the action of X rays on reproductive bodies (gametes).

X-ray films (radiographs), fluoroscopic scans, and isotopes are of great value in diagnoses. Some isotopes are radioactive, others are not. Various isotopes are used in therapy, others as tracers or to outline organs for contrast X-ray studies. Almost every organ within the body can now be explored through a form of radiation, making unnecessary many operations, including some exploratory surgery.

If your doctor sends you to a specialist for X rays, be sure the doctor who uses radiation on you is accredited by the American Board of Radiology. The person may be a radiologist, qualified to use X rays, radium, and radioactive substances for diagnosis and treatment, or he may be a roentgenologist, qualified to use only X rays for diagnosis and treatment.

This is no time to try to save money by having "pictures taken" by a technician with a year of on-the-job training. The doctor who specializes in radiology can interpret findings for your physician. This doctor will have his instruments in perfect working order, aim precisely the first time, and use patient-protecting shields or a collimator to confine the X-ray beam to the part of the body being exposed.

To help you identify tests for your records, the following descriptions of various types of diagnoses by radiation include mention of opaque substances when they are given:

1. Chest X-ray films are taken primarily to view the lungs; however, they also show the heart size and part of the rib cage. Once part of a routine checkup, they are now made only when necessary.
2. Bone X rays reveal fractures, malformations, or bone disorders.
3. Gall bladder X rays require a patient to take iodized tablets (unless allergic to seafood) and to omit fats from the diet the day before. Sometimes the radiologist will have the patient drink cream or eat rich food, then take more X rays when the food has reached the duodenum.
4. In fluoroscopy the patient is moved on a special table or he stands while a screen moves. The radiologist studies inner functions of the body, sometimes taking a series of X-ray still or moving pictures. The G.I. (gastrointestinal) series is an example of fluoroscopic scanning. (a) The upper G.I. examination re-

quires fasting for eight hours to prevent shadows cast by food. After the patient drinks a barium milkshake, the radiologist checks for ulcers, obstructions, or other conditions as the opaque barium passes through the organs. (b) Before the lower G.I. examination, castor oil and enemas clear the colon. A barium solution is used to enable the radiologist to see the colon under the fluoroscope and take X rays with the patient in various positions. Occasionally this is followed by an air-contrast study.

5. Heart trouble may be noted on simple X rays of the chest, but sometimes an opaque substance is injected to observe the heart and the blood vessels leading to and from the lungs. X-ray movies, called cine-angiograms, are taken for the cardiologist.

6. Bronchial tubes are X-rayed after iodized oil is inserted through the windpipe.

7. Kidneys, ureter, and bladder are X-rayed after a temporary dye is injected into a vein or introduced through the bladder.

8. Slipped disks can be identified by a radiology study after opaque iodine is inserted in the spinal canal.

9. The skull and brain are X-rayed to show possible bone fractures, contusions, or abnormalities. Other examinations include nuclear brain scans, air-contrast studies, and cerebral angiograms.

10. Breasts are X-rayed by mammography to show possible tumors. Occasionally radiologists can determine whether lumps are malignant or benign (cancerous or not).

11. Tomographs make one layer or part of the body clearly visible, blurring the surrounding areas.

Pregnant women are now rarely X-rayed because of possible damage to the fetus. Safe thermography can sometimes give needed information. Dental X rays should be avoided during early months of a pregnancy.

Radiation treatments by X rays, radium (gamma rays), or radioactive isotopes such as cobalt and cesium are now used only on malignant growths within the body. Before the hazards of too much radiation were known, X rays were used occasionally to treat tonsils, adenoids, glands in the neck, acne, arthritis, and other conditions. Fluoroscopy was used to see how shoes fit the feet. These procedures have been discontinued because it was found that cancer may develop in some persons as long as twenty to thirty years later. If you were treated by X rays many years ago, go back to that hospital for a checkup or see your physician immediately.

List X-ray studies made during recent years and the location of films or other information for your physician's reference. In many cases a series of X rays, taken over a period of years, will aid the doctor in diagnosis. When you visit specialists or change physicians, your records will help you guard against the excessive radiation to which many patients are subjected. However, new X rays may be needed from time to time, for the body is constantly changing.

Date	Body part X-rayed	Diagnosis and treatment	Information at

Date	Body part X-rayed	Diagnosis and treatment	Information at
_____	_____	_____	_____
		_____	_____
_____	_____	_____	_____
		_____	_____
_____	_____	_____	_____
		_____	_____
_____	_____	_____	_____
		_____	_____
_____	_____	_____	_____
		_____	_____
_____	_____	_____	_____
		_____	_____
_____	_____	_____	_____
		_____	_____
_____	_____	_____	_____
		_____	_____
_____	_____	_____	_____
		_____	_____
_____	_____	_____	_____
		_____	_____

My Electrodiagnoses

Recordings of various electrodiagnoses are made on graph paper. Best-known to most people are electrocardiograms (ECGs or EKGs) to measure heart action. Electrical currents in the brain, eyes, ears, muscles, stomach, etc., are measured when they could be significant in diagnosing a possible disorder.

Date	Test	Information at

My Chemistry and Physiology

Record all other tests on the physiology and chemistry of your body. Among the many tests you will want to include are: metabolism, glucose tolerance, cell specimens, bone marrow, biopsies, spinal fluid, Wassermann, hormones, smears, culture tests, bronchoscopy, proctoscopy, bacteriology, mucus, saliva, gastric juice.

Date	Test	Information at

Health Maintenance Organizations

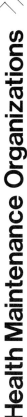

HMOs combine multiple screening tests, group practice, and health insurance through prepaid medical plans. Some have been operating successfully for years while others are in the experimental stages. Some sections of the country will not offer HMO plans until pilot projects have proved practical.

Generally, HMOs are affiliations of salaried physicians, specialists, nurses, and technicians. Members of HMOs pay, in advance, negotiated fees and obtain specified services at no further cost. Fees and services vary among HMOs and with individual patients' wants, e.g., single person or family coverage, routine and/or emergency care, inpatient/outpatient hospital services, home health services, diagnostic tests, dental care, psychiatric care.

Advocates of HMOs say that prepaid care motivates patients to come in for more frequent checkups and for earlier diagnoses and treatments of incipient disorders. Doctors are encouraged to practice preventive medicine to avoid emergencies, keeping down medical costs. They try to keep people well instead of simply treating the ill. It is reported that members of prepaid group plans spend fewer days in hospitals than the national average.

Note if you are a member of a Health Maintenance Organization:

HMO _____

Address _____

City, State _____

Phone _____

If you move and change to another Health Maintenance Organization:

HMO _____

Address _____

City, State _____

Phone _____

HMO _____

Address _____

City, State _____

Phone _____

For your own protection, copy prescriptions in this record so another doctor will not prescribe a medicine incompatible with one you are taking at the same time. Note when and why a medicine is discontinued and throw out any remaining. If you had adverse reactions to any drug before starting these records—even though you don't remember the dates, dosage, or strength—write the name or describe the medicine and what it was taken for and give your reactions under "Reason for discontinuing" on the following charts.

If the doctor does not record information on the next pages, you can do it from his prescription. The pharmacist's label seldom gives all the facts. Enter the trade or generic name for the drug. If it is a tablet or capsule that comes in more than one size, the strength is given in mg (milligrams), mcg (micrograms), gm (grams), gr (grains), or units. The number of tablets or capsules prescribed is shown as "#30" (or other number) or is given in roman numerals. A liquid or ointment may have a percentage of an active ingredient in a base, or it may be a compound identified only by product name.

The *Physicians' Desk Reference* gives physicians full information on over 2,500 brand-name drugs. This includes composition, action and uses, contraindications, precautions, side effects, adverse reactions, administration, and dosage. Many of the products are illustrated in this large book, published annually with updating supplements. When you get a new prescription, ask the doctor to show you or describe the medicine—tablet or capsule, size, shape, color, markings. Pharmacists have made mistakes. Most states require pharmacists to type the drug name on the label; if necessary, ask yours to do so.

The "signa" or "S" on the prescription form tells the dosage —how often you are to take the medicine. Copy the direction, "once a day" or the code: b.i.d. is twice a day, t.i.d. is three times a day, q.i.d. is four times a day, q.h. is every hour, q.d. is every day.

Be sure to find out *when* you are to take a medicine. Many drugs must be taken with or immediately after meals, some on an empty stomach, others one half hour before meals. Some must not be combined with alcohol, milk, fruit juice, antacids, or mineral oil.

In the lower left corner of the prescription form, the doctor gives refill instructions to the pharmacist. A check at "nonrep" means the prescription cannot be repeated (refilled). "P.r.n." is pro re nata, refill as needed. "Refill five times" means that, after the first prescription is filled, five refills are permitted by the doctor and by law within six months. If the doctor wants you to continue the medicine, you need a new prescription.

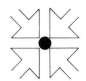

Transcriptions of Prescriptions

Prescribed For Me

Drug and strength	Dosage	Refills

Date started	Date stopped	Reason for discontinuing

Prescribed For Me

Drug and strength	Dosage	Refills

60

Date started	Date stopped	Reason for discontinuing

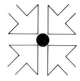

What I Do

During thorough examinations a doctor asks many questions, some of which you may think are none of his business. But they are! Your doctor is checking to find out whether your ailment, or tendency to one, may be due to your work, leisure-time activities, habits, or attitudes.

Possibly an illness may be your body's response to resentment, frustration, loneliness, worries, or other problems. A doctor needs to know whether you encounter occupational hazards such as dust, dampness, or chemical fumes—or if you are working under the stress of speed, noise, overcrowding, heavy responsibilities, interference from others, confusing directions, fear of dismissal, standing all day, or muscular strain. He may ask you to go through the motions used in your work or hobby to find out whether they may be causing bursitis, aching back, or tension in the neck, for instance.

When your doctor asks about your home and social life, it is not prying; the doctor is trying to find factors that may contribute to your less-than-best health. Illness is often called disease or disorder because a person does not feel ease or order in his life.

Occupations, present and past _____

_____

Recreations _____

Marital status _____

Occupations of spouse _____

Children, birth dates _____

How I Appraise Myself

Write: High, Middle, Low, or Never

Overeat	_____	**Exercise regularly**	_____
Try reducing diets	_____	**Enjoy recreations**	_____
Eat healthful foods	_____	**Feel energetic**	_____
Drink coffee, tea, colas	_____	**Am always tired**	_____
Drink alcohol	_____	**Feel bored, listless**	_____
Smoke tobacco	_____	**Sleep well**	_____

Smoke marijuana	_____	Am always prompt	_____
Try psychedelics	_____	Have good judgment	_____
Take amphetamines	_____	Have pleasant sex life	_____
Feel tense	_____	Feel self-confident	_____
Have anxieties	_____	Control my own life	_____
Know and like myself	_____	Am impulsive	_____
Resent some people	_____	Like to take risks	_____
Am patient, tolerant	_____	Am accident-prone	_____
Get along with others	_____	Adjust to situations	_____
Lead an active social life	_____	Plan each day's work	_____
Like my work	_____	Pray every day	_____
Yearn to succeed	_____	Take time for reflection	_____
Feel a drive to work hard	_____	Like a simple life	_____
Feel appreciated	_____	Get upset by bad news	_____
Take things easy	_____	Like to face facts	_____
Had strict parents	_____	Feel concern for others	_____
Had permissive parents	_____	Try to please people	_____
Worry about my family	_____	Often feel depressed	_____
Worry about money	_____	Like an orderly life	_____
Worry about my health	_____	Am a perfectionist	_____
Talk about health	_____	Feel hurried, frenzied	_____
Can tolerate pain	_____	Am swayed by emotions	_____
Am easily irritated	_____	Protest inequities	_____
Am sensitive to criticism	_____	Feel love and security	_____
Get in my own way	_____	Trust others	_____
Often feel frustrated	_____	Feel calm, content	_____
Fret at delays	_____	Enjoy living	_____

The body has several major systems engaged in communication, transportation, chemical transformation, storage, and protection. Each system performs a variety of separate functions, but all are linked. A previous or present disorder in part of a system could affect others. To review your knowledge of how body systems work, here are short, simplified descriptions. List disorders after each to let your doctors know.

Circulatory System

This is also called the cardiovascular system. "Cardio" refers to the heart and "vascular" to the blood vessels.

Your heart is as large as your clenched fist, whatever your body size. It is in the shape of a fist, with the broad knuckle end under the breastbone (sternum) and the narrow wrist end angled lower and to the left. Your left fist can demonstrate this.

A powerful muscular pump, the heart keeps blood circulating through about 120,000 kilometers (75,000 miles) of large and small blood vessels that, if placed end to end, would encircle the equator three times. An average adult has around 4.5 to 5.4 liters (5 to 6 quarts) of blood, but in the recycling a heart pumps 15,140 liters (16,000 quarts) each day.

The heart of an adult weighs around 224 grams (8 ounces), that of a baby less than 28 grams (1 ounce). With an atrium (auricle or upper storage room) and a ventricle on each side, there are four chambers in the heart.

The right atrium receives from the veins bluish-red blood with carbon dioxide and metabolic wastes. At every contraction the atrium pushes blood through the valve into the right ventricle which pumps it into the lungs to remove carbon dioxide and gather up oxygen from inhaled air. The left atrium receives oxygenated bright red blood from the lungs and impels it through the valve to the left ventricle. From this large chamber, blood is pumped through the aorta, arteries, and arterioles to the rest of the body.

Liquid plasma diffuses through the walls of blood vessels to carry oxygen and nutrients to the 60 trillion cells in the body and to take away their wastes. Arteries are strong, elastic, open tubes, unless clogged and hardened by disorders. Veins contain valves to prevent backflow and are squeezed by various muscles in the body to propel blood back to the heart.

When resting, an adult's heart averages 70 to 72 beats per

minute, though a range of 60 to 90 can be considered normal. A child's rate is 100 to 120 beats a minute. Heartbeats are felt as the pulse, with fingers over the large artery at the wrist. When an athletic teen-ager in excellent health exercises strenuously for at least ten minutes, his rate could go up to 200 beats a minute and, after a rest, go down to 40 or 50 beats.

Record anything on the heart and blood vessels that has bothered you. Include such things as varicose veins or a dull ache in the legs while walking.

Date	Cardiovascular problem	Treatment
————	————————————	————————————
————	————————————	————————————
————	————————————	————————————
————	————————————	————————————
————	————————————	————————————
————	————————————	————————————
————	————————————	————————————
————	————————————	————————————

Respiratory System

In volume, the body's greatest need is air—12,000 dry quarts a day. This is over 13,200 liters (375 bushels) to get oxygen, which is less than one fifth the volume of air. Oxygen is carried by the blood to every living cell in the body.

Inhaled through the nose at the rate of 12 to 20 (the average is 16 to 18) breaths per minute—more when exercising, less when sleeping—the air is cleaned, warmed, and moistened in the nasal passages. Air and food or liquid then take the same short tube to the epiglottis, a swinging door that separates the channels toward lungs and stomach. This anatomical arrangement lets you breathe through your mouth when swimming or when congestion blocks the nose, but it makes you "choke" and cough when you happen to inhale and swallow at the same time.

Air continues through the voice box (larynx) and the windpipe (trachea), both behind the Adam's Apple, down through the branched bronchi to the right and left lungs. Although the bronchioles (branches of the bronchi within the lungs) and the air sacs have muscles, the lungs themselves do not. Lungs are encaged by ribs in the chest cavity (thorax) and separated from the abdomen by the diaphragm, a muscle-membrane partition.

Breathing is controlled by nerve impulses to the diaphragm. As the diaphragm moves, the chest cavity and closely attached lungs expand. Air rushes in to fill the lung space. When the muscles in the diaphragm and between the ribs relax, air is forced from the lungs. With each breath cycle (inhalation and expiration) a pint of air is usually exchanged. Much more air remains in the lungs, which never collapse unless artificially opened.

Coughing can dislodge foreign particles and mucus. With chronic or severe attacks, see your doctor. Coughing could be a sign of pneumonia, chronic bronchitis, emphysema, lung cancer, or other disorders.

Although not part of the respiratory system, ears can be affected by sinus and nasal trouble. List here any ear disorders such as infections, injuries, impacted earwax, ear noises, hearing loss, abnormal growths, difficulty in maintaining body balance.

Colds: Frequent _____ . Seldom _____ . Never _____ .

If you smoke cigarettes: For how many years? _____ . How many per

   day? _____ .

If you quit smoking: When? _____ . After how many years? _____ .

Note here any persistent coughing, sinusitis, bronchitis, virus pneumonia, pneumonia, pleurisy, influenza, tuberculosis, or other respiratory and ear problems.

Date	Respiratory problem	Treatment
_____	_____	_____
_____	_____	_____
_____	_____	_____
_____	_____	_____
_____	_____	_____
_____	_____	_____
_____	_____	_____

Digestive System

What happens with the food you eat? Here's a simple explanation of the complex process known as digestion. It converts food into ever smaller and simpler components to build and repair the body's tissues and to supply energy. The process takes place in a tube 9 meters (30 feet) long. The tube widens, narrows, and curves into named parts with special functions.

The thought, smell, and sight of food starts the flow of salivary and gastric juices. Actual digestion begins in the mouth. As teeth grind the food, saliva pours in from three glands, and the tongue whips saliva with food to form a mush that's easy to swallow. Thorough chewing and mixing with saliva are the only direct controls a person has over digestion and are important because saliva supplies ptyalin, an enzyme that starts the digestion of starches.

The tongue and a sucking action at the back of the mouth move a chewed morsel of food (bolus) down the esophagus. Circular muscles contract and relax in waves (peristaltic action) to propel the food through the esophagus. At its base is a drawstring muscle, the cardiac valve, which controls the amount of food or liquid entering the stomach at one time. (The cardiac valve was named for its location and does not relate to heart action.)

Stomach muscles run in three directions to knead the food with gastric juice. A mixed-food meal is in the stomach from three to five hours. Liquids pass through quickly. Fats remain longest in the stomach but are not digested there.

Gastric juice contains hydrochloric acid and enzymes. Rennin coagulates milk. Pepsin converts meat and other proteins into a simpler, more soluble form. Although hydrochloric acid is corrosive, the stomach is lined with a mucous membrane that secretes mucus to protect it. Little of nutritional value is absorbed by the body from the stomach, but alcohol is. That's why its effects are felt quickly.

Food passes from the stomach through the pyloric valve into the horseshoe-shaped duodenum, the start of the small intestine. Here the digestive process changes. From physical churning and mixing with acid in the stomach, food is now subjected to more chemical activity and is drenched with alkaline fluids. Bile from the gall bladder and liver enters through the common duct. Pancreatic juice flows through its duct bringing enzymes: trypsin to change protein into amino acids, amylase to finish digesting carbohydrates, and lipase to split up fats so it and the bile can digest fats.

The liver is not actually a part of the digestive system. This large organ forms bile, but among other functions it stores glucose, manufactures or modifies elements, destroys uric acid, and detoxifies bacteria and harmful chemicals.

From the duodenum, the digesting food moves in peristaltic waves through the jejunum and ileum, 6 meters (20 feet) of small intestine. Enzymes and digestive juices continue their work of converting nutrients into fragments that can penetrate barriers to enter the body from the small intestine.

The material is semiliquid when it enters the large intestine. The primary purpose of the colon is to allow absorption of the moisture until the material is semisolid when it passes into the rectum, then moves down to the anus for excretion.

Do not clutter your records with temporary disturbances, but do list any that did cause or are now causing persistent discomfort or sharp pains. Include the liver, though it is interrelated with several systems, and the appendix.

Date	Digestive problem	Treatment
_____	_____	_____
_____	_____	_____
_____	_____	_____
_____	_____	_____
_____	_____	_____
_____	_____	_____
_____	_____	_____
_____	_____	_____

Nervous System

Without nerves one would be senseless and motionless. Nerves do not twitch, crawl, or tie themselves in knots. They flash signals in split seconds. For instance, if you drop a hammer on your foot, you won't feel pain until the brain identifies it. That's almost instantaneously, because messages travel up to 360 kilometers (225 miles) per hour.

Each nerve cell, called a neuron, has a body with receiving antennae (dendrites) and a sender or relayer (axon). Each neuron triggers a message to the next neuron in a chain reaction. Some neurons may be unbusy for a while, but they never go to sleep. Various estimates say there are from 10 to 30 billion neurons in the electrochemical network.

Ninety percent of the body's neurons are concentrated in the brain. Weighing only 1.36 kilograms (3 pounds), the adult brain is the most complicated and compact system ever created. It processes hundreds of items of information at the same time. In comparison, the most complicated computer is simply primitive.

The brain needs one fifth of the oxygen the blood supplies to the entire body. One faints if there is a temporary shortage and incurs brain damage or may die if the supply of oxygen is cut off for a few minutes. The brain also needs glucose for nourishment.

Nerves regulate involuntary or automatic activities such as heartbeat and digestion, and they communicate messages from the brain for voluntary activities such as reading or walking. Except for senses located in the head—sight, smell, taste, hearing, and touch to the head—all sensations and reactions travel via masses of nerve fibers in the spinal cord, a soft cable running through the vertebrae.

Birth defects, various infections, diseases, and injuries can affect the brain and nervous system. Although pain anywhere else in the body is apparent only when sensed in the brain, the brain does not feel pain within itself during surgery.

Enter problems directly related to the nervous system below. Such problems include amnesia or a severe bump on the head (no matter when it happened), tremors, jerking, rigidity, numbness, unsteady walk, convulsions, dizziness, fainting, nervous tics and spasms.

Date	Problem in nervous system	Treatment
_____	_____	_____
_____	_____	_____
_____	_____	_____
_____	_____	_____
_____	_____	_____
_____	_____	_____
_____	_____	_____

Endocrine System

Coordinated with the nervous system are glands that secrete hormones (chemical messengers) into the blood. They help to determine one's sex, physical characteristics, behavior, voice pitch, etc.

Except for the gonads (testes in men, ovaries in women), the endocrine glands are the same in both sexes. The *pituitary gland* is called the master gland because it breeds hormones that affect other endocrine glands. Little is known about the functions of the *pineal body*, a tiny gland also attached to the brain.

The *thyroid gland* looks like a butterfly in front of the windpipe. Using iodides supplied by the blood from food sources, the thyroid hormone affects metabolism, regulating the rate of oxygen use by most tissues of the body. Four bead-sized *parathyroid glands*, imbedded in the lobes of the thyroid gland, produce two hormones to regulate the supply of calcium in the blood. Below the thyroids is the *thymus*, a glandlike organ, that helps infants have some immunity to disease. It shrinks to almost nothing as one grows up.

The two triangular *adrenal glands* are in front of and above the two kidneys. They develop several hormones for "fight or flight" stress situations, influence metabolism, and supplement sex hormones. The large, elongated *pancreas gland* is below the stomach. It manufactures insulin and enzymes for the digestive system.

Gonad glands have two functions. One is to produce the hormones estrogen and progesterone, released into the blood to give feminine or masculine characteristics. The other generates reproductive seeds, ova in the female and sperm in the male.

Since a gland is defined as any secreting organ, there are around 100 in the body. The aforementioned glands are generally recognized as in the endocrine system, although some authorities question inclusion of the pineal body, thymus, and pancreas.

Date	Endrocrine problem	Treatment
____	_____	_____
____	_____	_____
____	_____	_____
____	_____	_____
____	_____	_____
____	_____	_____

The R-E System of Body Defense

Lining the blood-forming organs and blood vessels, the lymphatic system, and body cavities is the reticuloendothelial system of cells that ingest bacteria, dead tissue, and foreign matter. The medical term is used infrequently, but most persons are familiar with some of the system's disorders: anemia, hemophilia, leukemia, Hodgkin's disease, enlarged tonsils, swollen lymph nodes, thrombosis, edema.

Blood is manufactured in the red marrow of the bone. The red blood cells contain hemoglobin which carries oxygen from the lungs and returns with carbon dioxide and wastes. After four months red cells wear out; usable parts are salvaged by the spleen and liver.

Some types of white blood cells (leukocytes) are formed in the red marrow, others in the lymph nodes or spleen. The white cells can slip through blood vessels and rush to the site of an infection where they engulf and destroy bacteria. The number of white cells increases to meet an emergency. By testing the count, a doctor can find out whether there is an infection and how severe it is.

Platelets (thrombocytes) are tiny particles of basic cell material. They clump together to seal injured capillary walls and to clot blood after a cut to stop bleeding. These actions help defend the body, but in some disorders clots can grow large enough to obstruct blood vessels. Occasionally these thrombi loosen and travel to the lungs, causing pulmonary embolism.

The main purpose of the lymphatic system is to recapture the fluids supplied by blood vessels to moisten and nourish tissue cells. The system also picks up fat from the small intestine. Around 100 lymph nodes in the system act as filter traps for bacteria. When any of these swell, there is an infection that needs a physician's attention.

Note any instances of swollen tonsils or lymph nodes, edema, anemia, or blood clots and whether you are a hemophiliac.

Date	Problem in R-E system	Treatment

Genitourinary System

Blood and other body fluids are filtered through the intricate structure of the two kidneys around fifteen times a day. The kidneys extract impurities, water, and excess materials, including hormones, to form urine. In this way they regulate the composition of the fluids recycled to the body.

The kidneys are behind the abdomen, just below the rib cage, protected by the spine and large muscles in the back. From 170 liters of filtrated fluid, they concentrate around 1.4 liters of urine per day for an adult. The urine is collected in cuplike chambers in the kidneys; it then flows down the ureter tube into the bladder for temporary storage.

The average adult bladder can hold 0.5 liter (1 pint) of fluid. Fullness, the compression of pregnancy, cold weather, and stress, or irritation from alcohol, coffee, and spices affect the urge to urinate. A drawstring-type muscle (sphincter) at the bladder base opens, and neurons send the message to the brain. Normally, a person has voluntary control for a brief time over the opening of a second, lower sphincter leading to the urethra, the tube which extends from the bladder to the exterior. The female urethra is about 4 centimeters (1.5 inches) long. The male urethra is six times as long and passes through the prostrate gland to dispose of its secretions as well as urine.

Closely allied to the urinary system are some of the sexual organs. The gonads (testes and ovaries) are in the endocrine system. Although other reproductive organs are not described in this book, include any problems you have had with them here.

Date	Genitourinary problem	Treatment

72

SKELETON

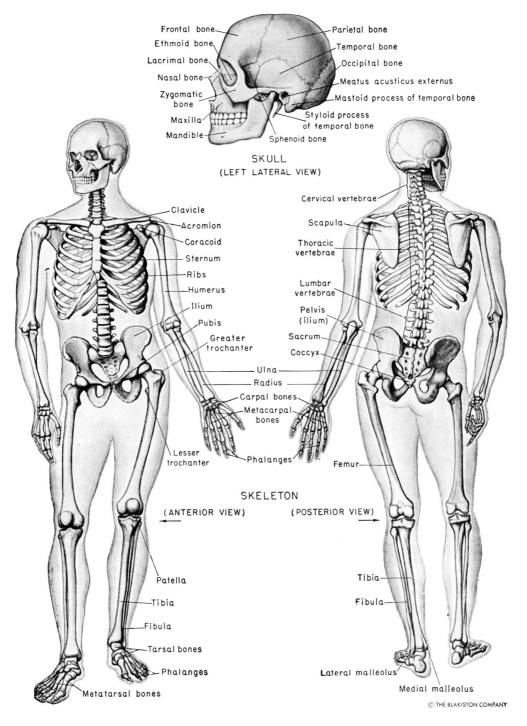

Frontal bone
Ethmoid bone
Lacrimal bone
Nasal bone
Zygomatic bone
Maxilla
Mandible

Parietal bone
Temporal bone
Occipital bone
Meatus acusticus externus
Mastoid process of temporal bone
Styloid process of temporal bone
Sphenoid bone

SKULL
(LEFT LATERAL VIEW)

Clavicle
Acromion
Coracoid
Sternum
Ribs
Humerus
Ilium
Pubis
Greater trochanter
Ulna
Radius
Carpal bones
Metacarpal bones
Lesser trochanter
Phalanges

Cervical vertebrae
Scapula
Thoracic vertebrae
Lumbar vertebrae
Pelvis (ilium)
Sacrum
Coccyx
Femur

Patella
Tibia
Fibula
Tarsal bones
Phalanges
Metatarsal bones

Tibia
Fibula
Lateral malleolus
Medial malleolus

SKELETON
(ANTERIOR VIEW) ⟵   ⟶ (POSTERIOR VIEW)

VISCERA

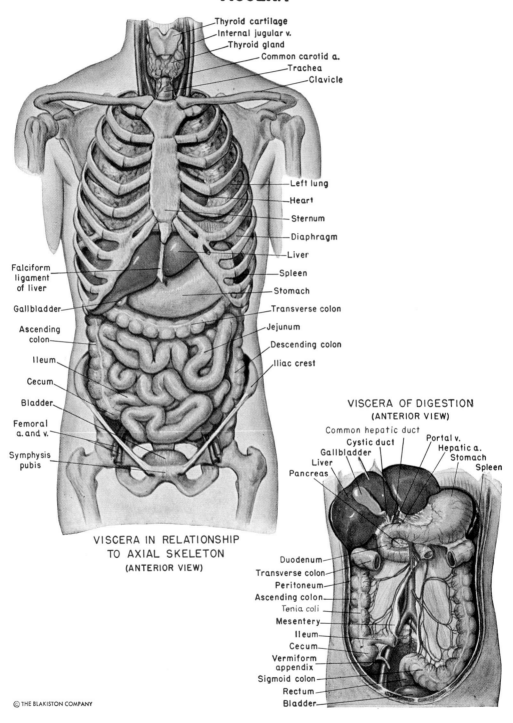

Thyroid cartilage
Internal jugular v.
Thyroid gland
Common carotid a.
Trachea
Clavicle

Left lung
Heart
Sternum
Diaphragm
Liver
Spleen
Stomach
Transverse colon
Jejunum
Descending colon
Iliac crest

Falciform
ligament
of liver

Gallbladder

Ascending
colon

Ileum

Cecum

Bladder

Femoral
a. and v.

Symphysis
pubis

VISCERA IN RELATIONSHIP
TO AXIAL SKELETON
(ANTERIOR VIEW)

VISCERA OF DIGESTION
(ANTERIOR VIEW)

Common hepatic duct
Cystic duct
Gallbladder
Liver
Pancreas

Portal v.
Hepatic a.
Stomach
Spleen

Duodenum
Transverse colon
Peritoneum
Ascending colon
Tenia coli
Mesentery
Ileum
Cecum
Vermiform
appendix
Sigmoid colon
Rectum
Bladder

MUSCLES

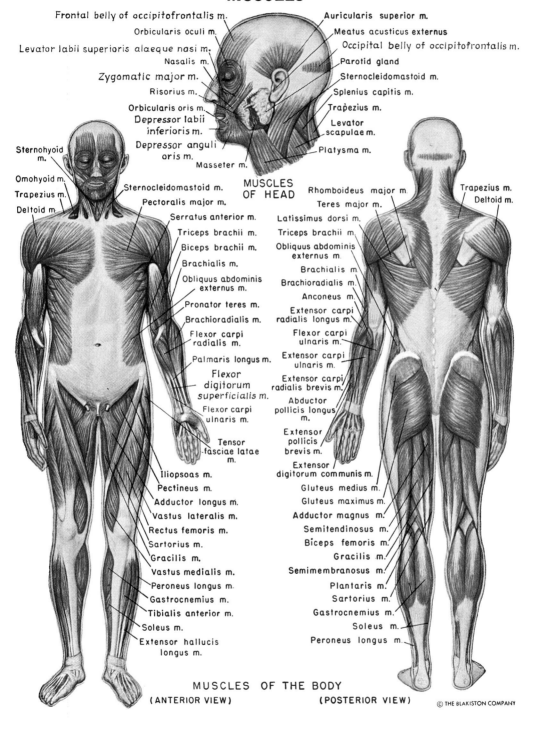

Frontal belly of occipitofrontalis m.

Orbicularis oculi m.

Levator labii superioris alaeque nasi m.

Nasalis m.

Zygomatic major m.

Risorius m.

Orbicularis oris m.

Depressor labii inferioris m.

Depressor anguli oris m.

Masseter m.

Auricularis superior m.

Meatus acusticus externus

Occipital belly of occipitofrontalis m.

Parotid gland

Sternocleidomastoid m.

Splenius capitis m.

Trapezius m.

Levator scapulae m.

Platysma m.

MUSCLES OF HEAD

Sternohyoid m.

Omohyoid m.

Trapezius m.

Deltoid m.

Sternocleidomastoid m.

Pectoralis major m.

Serratus anterior m.

Triceps brachii m.

Biceps brachii m.

Brachialis m.

Obliquus abdominis externus m.

Pronator teres m.

Brachioradialis m.

Flexor carpi radialis m.

Palmaris longus m.

Flexor digitorum superficialis m.

Flexor carpi ulnaris m.

Tensor fasciae latae m.

Iliopsoas m.

Pectineus m.

Adductor longus m.

Vastus lateralis m.

Rectus femoris m.

Sartorius m.

Gracilis m.

Vastus medialis m.

Peroneus longus m.

Gastrocnemius m.

Tibialis anterior m.

Soleus m.

Extensor hallucis longus m.

Rhomboideus major m.

Teres major m.

Latissimus dorsi m.

Triceps brachii m.

Obliquus abdominis externus m.

Brachialis m.

Brachioradialis m.

Anconeus m.

Extensor carpi radialis longus m.

Flexor carpi ulnaris m.

Extensor carpi ulnaris m.

Extensor carpi radialis brevis m.

Abductor pollicis longus m.

Extensor pollicis brevis m.

Extensor digitorum communis m.

Gluteus medius m.

Gluteus maximus m.

Adductor magnus m.

Semitendinosus m.

Biceps femoris m.

Gracilis m.

Semimembranosus m.

Plantaris m.

Sartorius m.

Gastrocnemius m.

Soleus m.

Peroneus longus m.

Trapezius m.

Deltoid m.

MUSCLES OF THE BODY

(ANTERIOR VIEW)   (POSTERIOR VIEW)

© THE BLAKISTON COMPANY

EYE

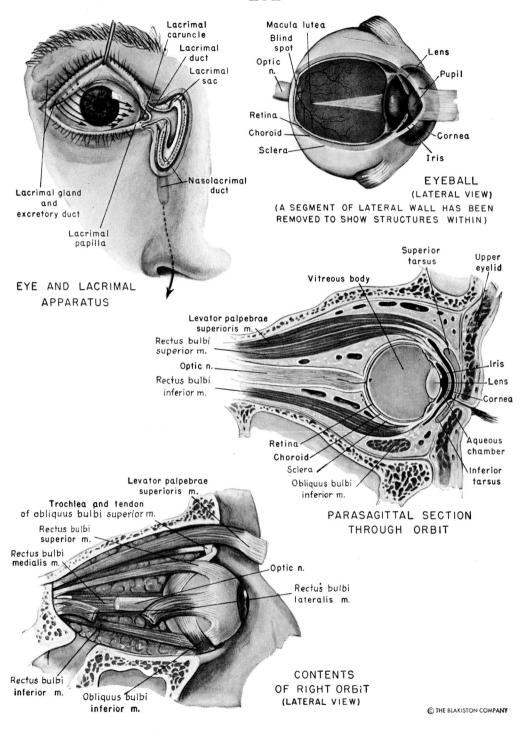

Lacrimal caruncle

Lacrimal duct

Lacrimal sac

Nasolacrimal duct

Lacrimal gland and excretory duct

Lacrimal papilla

EYE AND LACRIMAL APPARATUS

Macula lutea

Blind spot

Optic n.

Retina

Choroid

Sclera

Lens

Pupil

Cornea

Iris

EYEBALL
(LATERAL VIEW)
(A SEGMENT OF LATERAL WALL HAS BEEN REMOVED TO SHOW STRUCTURES WITHIN)

Superior tarsus

Upper eyelid

Vitreous body

Levator palpebrae superioris m.

Rectus bulbi superior m.

Optic n.

Rectus bulbi inferior m.

Iris

Lens

Cornea

Aqueous chamber

Inferior tarsus

Retina

Choroid

Sclera

Obliquus bulbi inferior m.

PARASAGITTAL SECTION THROUGH ORBIT

Levator palpebrae superioris m.

Trochlea and tendon of obliquus bulbi superior m.

Rectus bulbi superior m.

Rectus bulbi medialis m.

Optic n.

Rectus bulbi lateralis m.

Rectus bulbi inferior m.

Obliquus bulbi inferior m.

CONTENTS OF RIGHT ORBIT
(LATERAL VIEW)

Musculoskeletal System

Chemically aroused to action by nerves, the muscles work in teams, contracting to move body parts and relaxing for a return to position. In many areas of the body the muscles use bones for leverage and have the support of tendons (sinews). Tendons are tough bands of tissue joining muscles to bones and transmitting the force of the muscles to move the bones.

Bones are the most important factor in giving shape and support to the body. An adult has 206 distinct bones joined by tendons, ligaments, and other strong connective tissue. Bones are two thirds mineral and one third organic matter, omitting water content. They build and repair themselves and store minerals such as calcium. Most bones contain marrow that manufactures blood cells.

Bones are structured for weight bearing, organ protection, and range of motion needed. Correct posture, maintained by voluntarily controlled muscles, is important to avoid disorders including some types of headaches, disk trouble, and low back pain.

Each foot has 26 bones, 19 muscles, and over 100 ligaments—in a complicated assemblage of parts. Feet bear the body's weight, and if not working properly, your feet will hurt and cause discomfort in other parts of the body.

Among the musculoskeletal disorders for which you need to see a doctor are fractures, injured kneecap, "growing pains" in bones, arthritis, swollen joints, bone spurs, chronic bursitis, disk problems, frequently recurring low back pain, instability of hip joint or vertebrae, chronic muscle spasms, and painful stiffness without apparent cause. Note earlier and present disorders.

Date	Musculoskeletal problem	Treatment

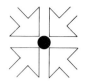

Visual problems affect about 130 million Americans. Half of all blindness is preventable.

Since eyes need extra careful care, why try to treat them yourself? Between regular checkups on possible need for corrective lenses or changes in prescriptions, see your eye doctor immediately for any of these conditions:

1. Injury to the eye from a foreign body, chemical, burn, cut, or blow.
2. Bacterial infections in the eyelash follicles (sties) or on the eyelids (blepharitis, with its itching, burning, swollen, and scaling eyelids).
3. Inflammatory redness in the white of the eye that may be due to a hemorrhage.
4. Pinkeye (conjunctivitis) from bacterial infection, allergy, or irritation.
5. Muddy change of color in the iris (the blue, hazel, or brown area around the dark pupil).
6. Overly tearful eyes or pus in the eyes.
7. Pain or discomfort in the eyes.
8. Lessened ability to move the eyes.
9. Blurred, cloudy, or diminished vision.
10. Eyes that can't adjust sufficiently to light changes or that ache in bright light.
11. Seeing nonexistent flashes of light or halos around lights.
12. Dimming or clouding of vision.
13. Distorted view of shapes and sizes.
14. Enlargement of the pupil of one eye.
15. A blind spot (scotoma) in the field of vision.
16. Preschool children should be examined for crosseye or "lazy eye" (amblyopia).
17. Protrusion of one or both eyes (which may be due to a thyroid problem or to an eye disease).

Who's who in eye care: An ophthalmologist or oculist is an M.D. who specializes in eye diseases and prescriptions for refractive errors (those which involve the bending of light rays). An orthokeratologist is an M.D. who is specializing in corrective contact lenses. An optometrist measures the degree of visual acuity and fits lenses. An optician makes eyeglasses or contact lenses.

Adjustment to contact lenses takes longer for new users, often two months, but you should be able to adjust to new lenses in spectacles in two days. Guard against errors by opticians who do not recheck but simply say, "Keep wearing them. You'll get used to them." Have your eye doctor check the lenses to make sure the prescription was ground correctly.

Occasionally, eye doctors err in writing prescriptions. One wrote "+1.25" instead of "−1.25" for the left lens. The patient asked the optician to check her previous prescription, but he kept records for only three years. At home she found copies of previous prescriptions which showed her left eye had always required a minus in the spherical correction. The ophthalmologist admitted his error, and the optician remade the lens. Note that plastic lenses, when put in large metal frames, tend to bend and conform to the frame shape.

Common refractive errors are:

1. *Hyperopia (farsightedness):* The image is focused behind the retina (membrane that receives the image).
2. *Myopia (nearsightedness):* The image is focused in front of the retina.
3. *Astigmatism:* Refraction varies in the eyeball, causing imperfect images or indistinct vision. Children with uncorrected astigmatism often get car-sick.

Prescriptions for glaucoma or other eye disorders

Date	Medication and strength	Directions

Rx for Refractive Errors (O.D. is the right eye. O.S. is the left eye)

Date_____. Dr._____

Type of lenses: Regular____. Bifocal____. Trifocal____. Contact ____.

		Spherical	Cylindrical	Axis	Prism	Base
Distance	O.D.					
	O.S.					
Add for Near	O.D.			Add for Intermediate	O.D.	
	O.S.				O.S.	

Date_____. Dr._____

Type of lenses: Regular____. Bifocal____. Trifocal____. Contact ____.

		Spherical	Cylindrical	Axis	Prism	Base
Distance	O.D.					
	O.S.					
Add for Near	O.D.			Add for Intermediate	O.D.	
	O.S.				O.S.	

Date_____. Dr._____

Type of lenses: Regular____. Bifocal____. Trifocal____. Contact ____.

		Spherical	Cylindrical	Axis	Prism	Base
Distance	O.D.					
	O.S.					
Add for Near	O.D.			Add for Intermediate	O.D.	
	O.S.				O.S.	

Date_____. **Dr.**_____

Type of lenses: Regular____. **Bifocal**____. **Trifocal**____. **Contact**____.

		Spherical	Cylindrical	Axis		Prism	Base
Distance	O.D.						
	O.S.						
Add for Near	O.D.			Add for Intermediate	O.D.		
	O.S.				O.S.		

Date_____. **Dr.**_____

Type of lenses: Regular____. **Bifocal**____. **Trifocal**____. **Contact**____.

		Spherical	Cylindrical	Axis		Prism	Base
Distance	O.D.						
	O.S.						
Add for Near	O.D.			Add for Intermediate	O.D.		
	O.S.				O.S.		

Date_____. **Dr.**_____

Type of lenses: Regular____. **Bifocal**____. **Trifocal**____. **Contact**____.

		Spherical	Cylindrical	Axis		Prism	Base
Distance	O.D.						
	O.S.						
Add for Near	O.D.			Add for Intermediate	O.D.		
	O.S.				O.S.		

Date_____. **Dr.**_____

Type of lenses: Regular____. **Bifocal**____. **Trifocal**____. **Contact**____.

		Spherical	Cylindrical	Axis	Prism	Base
Distance	O.D.					
	O.S.					

Add for Near	O.D.			Add for Intermediate	O.D.	
	O.S.				O.S.	

Date_____. **Dr.**_____

Type of lenses: Regular____. **Bifocal**____. **Trifocal**____. **Contact**____.

		Spherical	Cylindrical	Axis	Prism	Base
Distance	O.D.					
	O.S.					

Add for Near	O.D.			Add for Intermediate	O.D.	
	O.S.				O.S.	

Date_____. **Dr.**_____

Type of lenses: Regular____. **Bifocal**____. **Trifocal**____. **Contact**____.

		Spherical	Cylindrical	Axis	Prism	Base
Distance	O.D.					
	O.S.					

Add for Near	O.D.			Add for Intermediate	O.D.	
	O.S.				O.S.	

Proper home care of your teeth, plus regular visits to a dentist, can cut way down on dental difficulties. Yet 98 percent of Americans have had or will have such problems. Over 25 million have lost all of their teeth. Teeth are lost because of untreated cavities or as a result of gum disease, which affects two out of three people. Children and teen-agers often develop early symptoms of gum disease, and after age forty it accounts for 70 percent of the teeth lost.

Keeping teeth requires cleaning them, completely and often. Ideally, they should be cleaned after each meal, snack, or beverage. When that is impossible, as it is for most people, rinse your mouth well with water and clean teeth thoroughly at least once a day.

Brush teeth from the gumline to biting edge, concentrating on from one to three teeth at a time before moving on. Brush the chewing surfaces of back teeth in all directions to clean the fissures. Brush back and forth along the narrow crevice between teeth and gum edge, holding the brush at a forty-five-degree angle.

Each tooth has five sides that you can reach, so floss the sides between adjoining teeth with unwaxed dental floss every day. Use floss with a "threader" to reach under bridges or splints.

Thorough cleaning with floss and brushing at least once a day is necessary to remove plaque, a sticky film of saliva and bacteria (always present in the mouth) that feed on sugars and starches. The bacteria produce an acid that dissolves tooth enamel, causing cavities (dental caries). Bacterial plaque can also accumulate in the crevice between teeth and gums to irritate the gums.

Where plaque is not removed daily, it hardens into tartar or calculus. As this deposit builds up between teeth and gums, it separates teeth from the surrounding tissues. More bacteria invade the spaces. Gums become swollen and inflamed, often bleed. There may or may not be pus. Usually there is "bad breath." If not treated, the gum disease can destroy the gingival margin, periodontal membrane, cementum, and bone—all of which hold teeth firm.

At least every six months have your family dentist examine your teeth, gums, mouth, and jaws. The dentist or dental hygienist will give your teeth a thorough cleaning (prophylaxis) either by scraping or using an ultrasonic machine that vibrates plaque from teeth. Ask for directions on flossing your teeth correctly. Full-mouth X rays are usually needed every two to three years. When a few teeth pose problems, they may be X-rayed more frequently.

Depending on size and location of cavities, fillings can be of gold, silver alloy (amalgam), porcelain, or dental plastics. For crowns and caps, stainless steel is less expensive than gold; porcelain is baked onto metal for the visible sides.

Uneven permanent teeth should have orthodontics (straightening with braces) to prevent future problems that can be more expensive to treat. Straightening is usually started at around age thirteen, and braces are worn for about fifteen months. Some adults have had successful orthodontic therapy.

Who's who in dental care:

1. *Family dentist* checks regularly on the health of your mouth. In addition to cleaning and filling teeth, some are also experienced in straightening teeth, performing extractions, treating root canals and gum diseases, and making bridges and dentures.
2. *Pedodontist* cares for the teeth and mouths of children.
3. *Orthodontist* straightens teeth and corrects malocclusion so teeth will work together to cut, tear, crush, and grind food.
4. *Endodontist* does root canal work, treating infections in nerve or pulp chambers.
5. *Periodontist* treats diseases of the gums and other tooth-supporting structures.
6. *Oral surgeon* extracts teeth, sets fractures of jaw and facial bones, removes mouth tumors and tori (bony masses occasionally found on the tongue side of lower teeth).
7. *Oral pathologist* diagnoses diseases of the mouth.
8. *Prosthodontist* handles tooth replacement by removable or permanent appliances.

On the next page is a diagram of the thirty-two "permanent" teeth. The tooth numbers are identifications used by many dentists. The column of type uses these tooth numbers, names the teeth, and gives the average years of age when each erupts.

First, record below any treatment for straightening teeth, periodontics, jaw fractures, salivary glands, or the removal of tori, cysts, or tumors in the mouth.

Date	Treatment
_____	_____
_____	_____
_____	_____
_____	_____
_____	_____

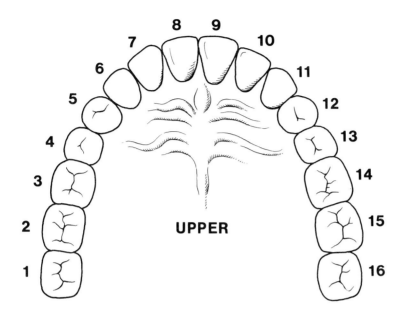

UPPER

32 "PERMANENT" TEETH

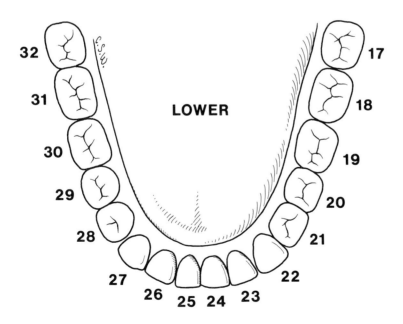

LOWER

81

1. **Wisdom tooth,** 17–21
2. **2nd molar,** 12–13
3. **1st molar,** 6–7
4. **2nd bicuspid,** 10–12
5. **1st bicuspid,** 10–11
6. **Cuspid,** 11–12
7. **Lateral incisor,** 8–9
8. **Central incisor,** 7–8
9. **Central incisor,** 7–8
10. **Lateral incisor,** 8–9
11. **Cuspid,** 11–12
12. **1st bicuspid,** 10–11
13. **2nd bicuspid,** 10–12
14. **1st molar,** 6–7
15. **2nd molar,** 12–13
16. **Wisdom tooth,** 17–21

17. **Wisdom tooth,** 17–21
18. **2nd molar,** 11–13
19. **1st molar,** 6–7
20. **2nd bicuspid,** 11–12
21. **1st bicuspid,** 10–12
22. **Cuspid,** 9–10
23. **Lateral incisor,** 7–8
24. **Central incisor,** 6–7
25. **Central incisor,** 6–7
26. **Lateral incisor,** 7–8
27. **Cuspid,** 9–10
28. **1st bicuspid,** 10–12
29. **2nd bicuspid,** 11–12
30. **1st molar,** 6–7
31. **2nd molar,** 11–13
32. **Wisdom tooth,** 17–21

Tooth　　　　　　　　**Dates and treatments**

1 _____

2 _____

3 _____

4 _____

5 _____

6 _____

7 _____

8 _____

9 _____

10 _____

11 _____

12 _____

13 _____

14 _____

15 _____

16 _____

17 _____

18 _____

19 _____

20 _____

21 _____

22 _____

23 _____

24 _____

25 _____

26 _____

27 _____

28 _____

29 _____

30 _____

31 _____

32 _____

The twenty baby teeth are identified in the same directions, but with letters. Average eruption times are given in months.

Tooth	Upper	Months	Tooth	Lower	Months
A	2nd molar	24-26	K	2nd molar	20-24
B	1st molar	13-15	L	1st molar	12-14
C	Cuspid	18-20	M	Cuspid	16-18
D	Lateral incisor	9-10	N	Lateral incisor	7-9
E	Central incisor	7-8	O	Central incisor	6-7
F	Central incisor	7-8	P	Central incisor	6-7
G	Lateral incisor	9-10	Q	Lateral incisor	7-9
H	Cuspid	18-20	R	Cuspid	16-18
I	1st molar	13-15	S	1st molar	12-14
J	2nd molar	24-26	T	2nd molar	20-24

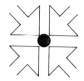

Do you really know the danger signals of heart attacks or strokes and of cancer, the leading life-takers? They've been widely published, yet most people are not aware of when to call an ambulance or see a doctor for a checkup. A survey showed two out of three people said they know, but only half of these "knowing" people could give more than one sign—and 27 percent could not identify a single signal of heart diseases. Thirty percent could not tell any of the seven warning signs of cancer, 17 percent could name one, and only 13 percent knew four or more.

Heart Attacks

Most persons who have one of the cardiovascular problems are able to live normally. But in 1973, 27 million Americans had cardiovascular diseases, responsible for more deaths than all other causes combined. Many deaths can be prevented if people recognize the early warnings and receive proper treatment immediately.

Cardiovascular diseases include atherosclerosis, coronary artery disease, stroke, high blood pressure, peripheral vascular disease, rheumatic heart disease, and congenital heart disease.

According to the American Heart Association*, the usual warnings of a heart attack are:

1. A heavy, squeezing pain in the center of the chest.
2. The pain may spread into the shoulder, arm, neck, or jaw.
3. Sweating.
4. Nausea, vomiting, and shortness of breath.

Strokes

A stroke occurs when something cuts off the brain's supply of blood, and it may affect any part of the body. Some persons recover quickly while others may not. The American Heart Association gives these possible causes:

1. Atherosclerosis in the arteries of the brain or neck may block the flow of blood.
2. A blood clot (thrombus) may form on the atherosclerosis, closing off the artery. This kind of stroke is a cerebral thrombosis.

*From *The Heart and Blood Vessels,* 1973, American Heart Association. Reprinted with permission.

3. A traveling blood clot (embolus) can stick in a small artery of the brain or neck. This kind of stroke is an embolism.
4. A weak spot in a blood vessel in the brain may break. This is a cerebral hemorrhage. (When the weak spot bulges, it is called a cerebral aneurysm.)
5. In rare cases, a brain tumor may press on a blood vessel and shut off the blood supply.

A "little stroke," the American Heart Association reports, warns that not enough blood is getting to the brain cells. It may be caused by a build-up of atherosclerosis or by a tiny blood clot partly blocking an artery. Signs of a little stroke may be:

1. A sudden, temporary weakness or numbness of the face, arm, or leg.
2. Temporary difficulty or loss of speech, or trouble understanding speech.
3. Brief dimness or loss of vision, particularly in one eye.
4. Double vision.
5. Unexplained headaches or a change in the kind of headaches you get.
6. Temporary dizziness or unsteadiness.
7. A recent change in personality or mental ability.

High-risk factors for strokes and heart diseases include cigarette smoking, overweight, diabetes, stress, hypertension, high cholesterol level in the blood, and lack of exercise to stimulate circulation and exercise the heart muscles.

Cancer

Around 222,000 American lives are saved each year through early detection and treatment of cancer, according to the American Cancer Society's estimate for 1975.* Yet 1,000 persons a day die from cancer.

Any of these seven warning signals of cancer should send you to a doctor for a checkup:

1. Change in bowel or bladder habits.
2. A sore that does not heal.

*Information from the American Cancer Society's '75 *Cancer Facts and Figures* © used with permission.

3. Unusual bleeding or discharge.
4. Thickening or lump in breast or elsewhere.
5. Indigestion or difficulty in swallowing.
6. Obvious change in wart or mole.
7. Nagging cough or hoarseness.

Notice that the word "caution" is spelled, when reading downward the first letter of each signal. And caution is the attitude to take toward cancer. Why be a fatalist, worrier, or neglecter? Practice the seven safeguards urged by the American Cancer Society:

1. Lung: Reduction and ultimate elimination of cigarette smoking.
2. Colon-Rectum: Proctoscopic exam as routine in annual checkup for those over forty.
3. Breast: Self-examination as monthly female practice.
4. Uterus: Pap test for all adult and high-risk women.
5. Skin: Avoidance of excessive sun.
6. Oral: Wider practice of early detection measures.
7. Basic: Regular physical examination for all adults.

Typically, cancer begins as a localized disease—on the surface of the skin or of the uterus, on the lining of the mouth, stomach, intestines, bladder, bronchial tube, or in the lining of a duct in the breast, prostate gland, or elsewhere. For a time cancer cells are visible only under a microscope. After invading the underlying tissue, they grow into an intact mass. As long as they remain where the disease started, they are localized and more readily treated.

Because early cancer is usually painless, one could have it unknowingly. Because some cancers grow and spread slowly but others develop rapidly, don't wait for your regular annual physical examination if you have any of the seven warning signals or are in a high-risk group. Have a cancer checkup which will include: (1) your medical history and (2) examinations of (a) skin, (b) head and neck, including mouth and throat, (c) chest, including an X ray, (d) abdomen, (e) colon and rectum, including proctoscopy, (f) blood, (g) urine. Also, men should have a prostate examination and women a Pap test and examination of the pelvic area and of the breasts by palpation (touch). For some patients physicians may also order mammography (breast X rays) or sputum cytology (laboratory tests on coughed-up matter).

Alcoholism

Over 10 million alcoholics in the United States make this disease too common. Alcoholism is more dangerous than other problems summarized in this chapter, for alcohol kills. It is a factor in half of the traffic fatalities each year. It can kill when taken with narcotics, sedatives, antihistamines, or some other drugs.

Alcohol kills slowly by causing or increasing health problems such as malnutrition, pellagra, gastritis, ulcers, gastroenteritis, cirrhosis of the liver, pancreatitis, pneumonia, nerve degeneration, and brain changes. It can increase heartbeats and blood pressure.

Only 5 to 10 percent is excreted. Alcohol is absorbed directly into the blood where it remains for about five hours. Generally, blood levels of 100 to 200 milligrams (mg) of alcohol per 100 milliliters (ml) of blood produce a feeling of euphoria. From 200 to 300 mg cause depression and loss of muscle coordination. Overuse of alcohol reduces the automatic control of breathing and heartbeat, and death often occurs with over 500 mg of alcohol in 100 ml of blood.

While still employed, alcoholics cost businesses $15 billion a year. The leading drug problem in the United States, alcoholism is recognized as a disease. Various treatments are available, and cures have been effective in 50 to 80 percent of the cases, depending upon individual motivation. For information write to National Council on Alcoholism, 1101 17th St., N.W., Washington, D.C. 20036.

Common Colds

Common colds are highly contagious, spreading quickly through home, school, office, or plant. Not only are the viruses airborne from sneezing, coughing, and tossing soiled tissues into wastebaskets, but they are also left on everything touched after nose-blowing. Handshakes spread contagion even further.

A study sponsored by the National Institute of Allergy and Infectious Diseases showed that chilling, overheating, or exposure to cold or damp weather have little effect on the development or seriousness of a cold.

Although emotional problems can help induce respiratory symptoms, 100 viruses have been identified with colds. The incubation period is eighteen to forty-eight hours. Young children often have a slight fever; adults rarely do. Distressing symptoms can be relieved by antihistamines or other cold products, but most of these should not be taken by anyone with a chronic illness such as

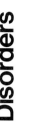

glaucoma and hypertension or with heart, circulatory, thyroid, or kidney trouble. A cold usually lasts from four to ten days unless complications develop. Sinusitis, laryngitis, bronchitis, sore throat, or coughing that lasts over two days may require a doctor's care.

Coughing that produces sputum removes mucus and dust irritants from the bronchial tubes and lungs. It should not be suppressed unless it prevents sleeping or strains the heart. With whooping, paroxysmal (sudden, uncontrollable, recurring), or smoker's cough, see your physician.

Here's how to distinguish the common cold from flu (influenza). Flu starts abruptly with chills, fever, aches and pains all over, headache, weakness, and loss of appetite. There may or may not be respiratory symptoms—stuffy nose, scratchy throat, unproductive cough. With the common cold, bed rest is desirable, though considered an indulgence. With the flu, you won't want to get out of bed until the day after your temperature returns to normal.

Backaches

Seven million people are treated each year for backaches, and seven times as many have them. A medical textbook lists 100 causes, and a clinic's survey notes twenty-eight different causes. Common backaches stem from poor posture while standing, sitting, or sleeping, from emotional tensions, arthritis, and lack of exercise to strengthen back muscles. Muscles are often sent into a spasm when lifting or pushing an object improperly.

Though onset of pain is sudden, the relaxing of muscles takes time, heat, massaging, and stretching. Usually pain subsides while affected muscles are at rest—but don't immobilize them. A structural weakness, whether congenital (existing from birth) or produced by bad habits, puts a chronic strain on the back. Abnormal curvature of the spine develops gradually. Discomfort worsens with fatigue, lessens when lying on a firm surface and with physiotherapy.

Persistent or recurring backaches may be referred pain from disorders in the stomach, intestines, pancreas, rectum, uterus, or prostate. Have your doctor check for those or for a ruptured disk, infection, bone fracture, or muscles too weak to support the torso.

Headaches

Transient headaches are usually related to tension, eyestrain, congestion in the nose or sinuses, fever, fatigue, hurry, boredom, hunger, chemical fumes, or too much alcohol, smoking, or rich food. When causes are eliminated, these headaches disappear. Tension headaches, the most common, are relieved by massaging the neck muscles, rolling the head, applying heat, or lying down. An example of a psychogenic headache is the headache one blames on eyestrain at work—and then one manages to watch television at home.

If headaches are frequent or constant, they may signal post-traumatic or organic disorders. Observe and record the nature of the pain, severity, location, frequency, and duration. See your physician, who may refer you to a neurologist for various tests.

Migraine headaches may have emotional, vascular, or biochemical causes—or a combination of these. Untreated, an attack may last for several hours or days. Make notes on your feelings (restlessness, irritability, etc.) before onset, the effects on your vision, the nature and location of pain, and whether you had chills or nausea. Take your notes and this health records book to your doctor. He can help you with therapeutic measures such as drugs, injections, or diets.

Depression

Depression is the leading untreated disorder. Each year around 20 million adults endure depressions but think nothing can be done for them. Symptoms are lethargy (unhealthy drowsiness, indifference to people, lack of desire to participate in activities), low spirits (sadness, melancholy, dejection, occasionally despair), anhedonia (lack of pleasure in doing something that ordinarily is enjoyable). Some individuals have delusions of persecution, hypochondria, guilt feelings, obsessive-compulsive behavior, hallucinations, or suicidal tendencies. The mental state is often accompanied by dry mouth, loss of appetite, constipation, insomnia, impotence, or decreased menstrual flow.

Factors in depression may be biochemical, electrolytic, or genetic. Doctors can help identify the cause and treat it so the person can again enjoy living.

An allergy is a hypersensitive reaction in some individuals to a substance (allergen) which does not bother other people. For example, pollen in the nose of one person will simply elicit a sneeze. Someone allergic to that pollen will have sneezing bouts, swollen nasal passages, and watery discharges from nose and eyes.

Half the population has occasional allergic reactions, while 10 percent have chronic or subacute problems. A tendency to hypersensitivity can be inherited, though the same allergies will not necessarily be present. White blood cells, in allergic people, will not engulf and destroy the particular allergen. Multiple sensitivities are usual; however, a person may be sensitive to only one substance. A first contact may not cause trouble, but repeated exposures often cause increasingly severe reactions. Emotional upsets occasionally play a role in allergies but do not cause them.

If an attack is acute, such as bronchial asthma, see a doctor immediately for treatment. He will instigate the search for external or internal causes. Blood tests are being developed to determine a few allergies, but doctors generally rely on skin testing. You cannot be skin tested for everything, so you will want to keep careful, detailed records to find clues. In most cases the detection of allergens requires more work by the patient than by the doctor—at least if you want to save your skin, money, and time. When you have found some suspects, take samples of the possibly offending substances, where feasible, to the doctor for skin tests. Cross off those found to be harmless.

Skin tests used to determine inhaled or contact allergens and in diagnosing and regulating therapy for some systemic diseases:

1. For patch tests the suspected substance is placed on paper or gauze and taped to the skin for twenty-four or forty-eight hours, unless removed earlier because it irritates the skin.
2. In scratch tests the skin surface is "torn," not cut, to avoid drawing blood. Possible allergens are applied to the scratches.
3. For intradermal tests syringes with fine needles inject each substance.
4. For indirect skin tests blood is drawn from a patient, centrifuged, and tested on a nonallergic person.

Contact Dermatitis

This is the cause of 75 percent of all occupational diseases. Symptoms include inflammation, itching, wheals (small acute swellings), rash, blisters, swelling, oozing, crusting, and scaling. They may not appear until two to four days after exposure.

If your skin reacts to any substance, try to trace the offender. When the allergen is identified, avoid further contact with it. If this is impossible, you may wish to have desensitization treatments—a series of subcutaneous (under the skin) injections of an extract of the allergen, in gradually increasing doses. If a person reacts adversely to the previous injection, dosage is adjusted. The frequency and number of treatments needed vary with each person's degree of sensitivity.

An important clue to finding an allergen may be the location and shape of the initial irritation such as the wrist under a watchband or waistline under elastic. If the inflammation followed the use of a new product, the ingredient list on the package may enable an allergist or a dermatologist to make fewer tests to find the offending agent. However, the Food and Drug Administration does not require the listing of basic ingredients on certain similar products. The setting of "standards of identity" does not help consumers. The doctor may need to get the complete list from the Poison Control Center, described in the "Crises" section of this book.

Note any changes in your customary contacts to do a preliminary finding. These are major suspects for the various body areas:

1. *Head and neck:* Cosmetics, shaving preparations, hair colorings, permanent wave solutions, nail polish on fingertips that touch the face, lipstick colorings, perfumes and colognes, propellants in hair sprays, jewelry, furs, pollens, dusts.

Suspects: _____

_____

_____

_____

2. *Torso:* Clothing—wool, silk, leather, fur, synthetic fibers, finishes, elastic, metals (especially nickel). Also deodorants, antiperspirants, and bath preparations.

Suspects: _____

_____

_____

_____

3. *Legs and feet:* Clothing, leather or plastic shoes, plants such as ragweed and poison ivy, oak, or sumac.

Suspects: _____

_____

_____

4. *Hands and wrists:* Any of the preceding. Also detergents, other cleansers, bleaches, polishes, chrysanthemums, primroses, white pine, balsa, kapok, a host of industrial chemicals, and handling citrus fruits, onions, celery, or other edibles. Because household products are often implicated, try narrowing the field of suspects. Each week wear cotton-lined rubber gloves only when using one or a group of products with similar ingredients to see whether the skin improves. Try soapless cleaners or oil and water to wash your hands and bathe. The culprit may be the perfume or alkali in bar soap.

Suspects: _____

_____

_____

_____

_____

_____

"Hypoallergenic" means low in known allergens. Cosmetics and toiletries so described are safer to use by a person with allergic tendencies, but no ingredient or combination can be guaranteed to be safe for everyone.

Inhaled Allergens

Prime suspects are pollen, mold, fungus, dust, pesticides, animal dander, insect excretions, smoke, or products with strong odors such as perfume and paint. Also various chemicals, especially when sprayed.

1. Describe allergic symptoms: _____

_____

2. Date and time symptoms began: _____

3. General environment on that date and the previous date. Get data from weather broadcast, newspaper, or local weather bureau:

Temperature range _____   **Pollen count** _____

Humidity _____   **Mold count** _____

Wind velocity _____   **Pollution** _____

Wind direction _____   **Precipitates** _____

With this information and some checking, you may find, for example, the southeast wind was blowing pollen from timothy grass, or fields to the west were crop-dusted with a pesticide. Note your findings:

_____

_____

_____

_____

4. Personal environment shortly before onset of symptoms. Moving or changing jobs will require a larger-scale investigation, but most individuals need note only what was different, not customary.

a. Where were you? E.g., flower market, farm, restaurant. If you were in an industrial plant, note the area, because 100,000 substances with possible allergens are used in industries.

_____

_____

_____

b. What did you do? E.g., cleaned a storage room, petted a friend's dog, painted the garage, picked up dry cleaning.

_____

_____

_____

c. What substances were different at home or business? E.g., a

93

bouquet of mums, dahlias, carnations (all in the ragweed family), a new article of clothing, or a new fragrance or furniture polish.

_____

_____

_____

Insect Allergens

If you have ever had an allergic reaction to the venom in a sting from a bee, hornet, wasp, yellow jacket, or fire ant, you should have injections to desensitize you. Future stings will have greater effect and may be fatal unless medication is given _immediately_. Until you are desensitized keep the allergy on your "Emergency?" page and carry an emergency kit. Wear an ID neck tag or bracelet noting your problem and the emergency measures required for treatment.

Insects, allergic reactions: _____

_____

_____

Date desensitizations started _____ . Dated completed _____ .

Mosquitoes and various kinds of flies bite. Most people have only minor irritations or become immune to their bites. However, the bits of lice, bedbugs, and some other ants may start allergic reactions in a few individuals and may require desensitization.

Drugs, Serums

If allergic to any of the medications commonly used in emergencies, these were entered in the "Emergency?" pages and you should wear an ID bracelet or neck tag. If you had adverse reactions to any other drugs or serums before keeping "Transcriptions of Prescriptions," they were entered in that section.

Because sensitivities are often due to genetic defects, help guard yourself against them from drugs you have not yet tried by telling your doctor about those listed in the "Maybe in My Genes" section. These are medications that have caused reactions to anyone in your family—in your blood line only, not your in-laws.

94

Physical Allergies

These are caused mainly by heat, cold, pressure, mechanical irritation, light and other radiations. Protect yourself from them. Ask your doctor whether antihistamine or adrenocortical therapy might relieve your symptoms.

Food Allergies

Individuals sensitive to inhalants may get attacks of bronchial asthma from smelling the food when it is being cooked or served, but usually a reaction comes only from eating the food. Symptoms occur within twenty-four hours and include hives, rash, indigestion, and nausea. If you or your children dislike any food intensely, this may be self-protective, indicating a possible allergy to be checked.

Digestive upsets do not always signify allergies to certain foods. Some may be due to animal diseases or chemicals given animals, to pesticides used on plants, to preservatives, seasonings, and colorings, or to improper processing or cooking of foods.

The most common food offenders are strawberries, oranges, seafood, chocolate, nuts, wheat, oatmeal, eggs, milk, and pork. Ham and bacon are changed in the curing process. Whatever is found to be an allergen to you should be avoided in all foods containing it: e.g., milk, eggs, and wheat flour are used in many foods. Flu vaccines prepared from fertilized eggs should not be taken by anyone sensitive to egg protein.

One way to trace food allergens is with a food diary. Keep a chart with foods listed at the left and dates across the top. Check all foods eaten each day for a month and note any reactions. By varying your menu, you may find out what foods are guilty. If you cannot and symptoms occur frequently, your doctor will give you the restricted food-elimination diet to help determine the offenders.

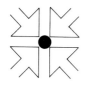

An adult is wrapped in an average of 20 square feet (1.8 square meters) of skin that weighs 7 pounds (3.15 kilograms). The skin not only protects the rest of the body from most external abuses but also serves in the sense of touch, as a temperature and fluid control, and as a warner of internal disorders.

Unlike other organs, the skin is readily observable. A skin specialist (dermatologist) or physician has direct access for diagnosis and local (topical) treatments. You can see when something is wrong and attend to the little problems that affect its health.

This simplified drawing of a magnified cross-section of skin shows its main components.

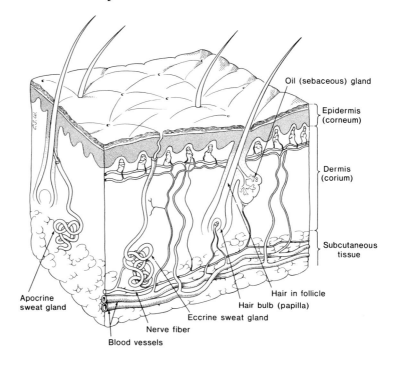

Oil (sebaceous) gland
Epidermis (corneum)
Dermis (corium)
Subcutaneous tissue
Hair in follicle
Hair bulb (papilla)
Eccrine sweat gland
Apocrine sweat gland
Nerve fiber
Blood vessels

What's in the Skin

The epidermis has several layers of cells. New cells germinate in the lowest layer and move to the surface in twenty-eight days, losing life en route. When they reach the outermost (horny) layer, the cells are dead and shed. This is a continual process, giving a new surface to your skin every four weeks.

The dermis contains tiny muscles, nerve fibers, and blood vessels so minute there are about 15 feet (4.5 meters) in 1 square inch (6.45 square centimeters) of skin. The hair shafts and oil and sweat glands originate here. Below the dermis, in varying thickness, is the subcutaneous tissue of resilient and fatty substances that cushion and insulate.

The 2 million coiled sweat glands are of two types. Eccrine glands are located almost everywhere on the body except the lips. To dispel excess heat from the body, they can secrete up to two quarts of dilute salt water a day. This evaporates when it reaches the skin surface, except in high humidity.

Apocrine sweat glands open into hair follicles in the under-arm and genital areas. The fluid they produce has no odor until it is decomposed by bacteria. Deodorants nullify the odor. Antiperspirants act within twelve hours to close the follicle openings for a day or two and have deodorant ingredients.

Sebaceous glands excrete oil into hair follicles. The oil (sebum) lubricates the hair and skin to keep natural moisture in them. Chemicals in sebum help maintain a healthy skin's slightly acid surface. A somewhat alkaline skin film is thought to increase susceptibility to infections and fungus. Oil glands are in all body skin except the palms and soles. They are most numerous on the face, neck, chest, and shoulders—all acne-prone areas.

Hair grows from almost all human skin except palms and soles, though it is not noticeable on most of the body. Hair cells form in the root bulb and cornify as they push up the slanting hair shaft to the skin surface. The hair you see is not a living substance; it is mostly keratin, a chemical. So are fingernails and toenails, hard and some-what flat plates of horny matter. The living part of a nail is beyond the half moon, in the matrix under the digital skin. Fingernails grow three times as fast as toenails. Hair on the scalp grows at the average rate of one third inch per month. Each individual hair rests from growing at different intervals so that about 5 percent of all strands are inactive at any one time.

Common Skin Problems

Dry skin: Sun, wind, water, heat, and air-conditioning draw from the skin the natural moisture that makes it soft and flexible. Oil in some form is needed to hold moisture in the skin surface. Many persons also need to add moisture to their skin. Lotions, creams, and oils used in baths or on wet skin will rehydrate the skin and guard against moisture loss.

Oily skin, acne: At puberty, the oil glands in the skin are stimulated to produce excess oil. If not removed frequently, the oil can combine with old skin cells and plug the outlet. Exposed to air, the plug darkens to become a blackhead (comedo). When bacteria invade the plug, it develops into a pimple which becomes a pustule if not treated. As more oil is produced, pressure builds up. If it ruptures the gland, oil and bacteria seep into the surrounding skin tissue, producing a cyst which should be treated by a skin specialist.

From 80 to 90 percent of all teen-agers have varying degrees of acne. Most outgrow it when their endocrine systems stabilize, though some persons have excessively oily skin with occasional break-outs all of their lives.

Take care of acne skin to avoid psychic trauma and permanent scarring. Wash skin thoroughly at least twice a day with a soap that contains drying ingredients such as sulfur. Apply a local preparation to dry up, unplug, and peel off blackheads, pimples, and pustules. Do not pick at or squeeze any blemish; that enlarges the problem. If acne is severe or you are impatient to have a clear complexion, consult a dermatologist.

Tetracycline is widely prescribed for acne cases, but antacids and milk or milk products reduce the ability of the body to absorb the drug. Iron (ferrous sulfate), taken by many teen-age girls, also interferes with the absorption of tetracycline. If iron tablets are necessary to avoid iron-deficiency anemia, ask the doctor for another prescription for acne or use products applied to the skin only.

Dandruff: Dandruff, or seborrheic dermatitis, is an excessive oiliness of the scalp apparent in oily scales and crusts. Using a shampoo containing zinc pyrithione, sulfur and salicylic acid, or selenium sulfide, leaving the lather on the head for five minutes, usually brings dandruff problems under control. If stronger treatment is necessary, therapeutic shampoos or lotions that also contain tar are left on the scalp all night and shampooed out in the morning. Untreated dandruff could aggravate acne or cause inflammation on the eyelids (blepharitis) or external ear (otitis).

Itching: Itching, or pruritus, may be local or general. Although it is instinctive to scratch, try not to. It just starts an itch- scratch cycle that accentuates the itching and may break the skin. Remove any local irritant such as woolen or rough-textured clothing. Use hand lotion or cream if itching is caused by dry skin. If caused by the bite of an insect to which you are not allergic, apply alcohol, camphor spirits, menthol, calamine lotion, glycerin, olive oil, or zinc oxide.

Because heat aggravates itching, take lukewarm baths. To relieve generalized itching, soak for 10 to 20 minutes in a tub of water into which you've mixed one of these: (1) 1 to 2 ounces (28 to 56 grams) of bath oil. (2) One cup colloidal oatmeal, available at drug stores. Sprinkle the powder into the tub under the faucet while water is running full force. (3) A thin paste of two cups of corn starch stirred with cold water. (4) One to two cups of baking soda. If itching persists despite your care, see a doctor, since itching is a symptom of several systemic diseases or may indicate the start of psoriasis or other skin disorder.

Heat rash or prickly heat: This condition (also known as miliaria) is due to a blocking of sweat ducts. Perspiration cannot reach the skin surface and evaporate. Heat rash may be caused by long contact with wet compresses, diapers, adhesive tape, too much clothing, or the sun. Symptoms are itching and pinpoint bumps—pale if the obstruction is near the surface, red if deeper. The rash disappears in hours or days in a dry, cool environment.

Excessive perspiration: Hyperhidrosis, when it appears on palms and soles, may be helped by: drying powder, soap containing sulfur and salicylic acid, or a solution with aluminum chloride or potassium permanganate. If the sweating is all over the body, is not due to a fever, or does not subside after a fever, see a physician.

Sun sensitivity: Skins vary greatly in their reaction to the sun. They do or don't tan, burn, freckle, blotch, blister, or break out in hives or an itchy rash. A combination of sun and substances on or in the skin can produce an unwanted effect. The individual may be using a fragrance containing oil of bergamot or taking a medication such as an antibiotic, sulfa drug, tranquilizer, barbiturate, or salicylate. People with certain diseases can have skin problems when exposed to sun. Too much sun-tanning will make a healthy skin look leathery and prematurely aged. Sunburn damages the skin. Overexposure to the sun is the leading cause of skin cancer, with 110,000 cases a year. Light-skinned persons are most susceptible. Staying out of the sun from 11 A.M. to 2 P.M. and using sunscreen preparations help but will not completely protect the sun-sensitive.

Poisonous substances: If your skin comes in contact with dangerous chemicals or radioactive material, wash skin immediately and thoroughly. Many poisons are quickly absorbed through the skin.

Skin pigmentations: Mistermed as liver spots, *lentigenes* are distinguished from freckles by their irregular shapes. They are level with the skin surface, whereas *keratoses* are flat-top growths that may be either scaly or smooth and shiny. Watch keratoses; some may be precancerous. If they thicken, roughen, form crusts, or bleed, see a physician. *Common moles* are raised clumps of pigmented cells, seldom dangerous unless irritated. If any start to grow fast or to bleed, have them checked. *Warts* (verrucae) are slightly contagious and can spread on a person and to others. Doctors remove warts with chemicals, electrodesiccation, excision, or freezing with liquid nitrogen.

Cold sores, fever blisters (herpes simplex Type I): Calamine lotion or spirits of camphor can dry up oozing lesions, and zinc oxide helps cracked ones. Doctors prescribe antibiotic pills or salves which also lubricate. If the virus should infect eyes, it will threaten vision; see a doctor immediately. Note: Do not confuse this with herpes zoster (shingles), which has blisters along a nerve route, or with herpes simplex Type II, which causes genital infections.

Boils: Boils can be brought to a "head" with hot packs, but if they don't open and drain by themselves, have a doctor care for them.

Chafing: Chafing is caused by warmth, moisture, and the friction of two opposing skin surfaces rubbing together. A frequent site is on the inner side of the thighs. Talcum and loose clothing relieve it.

Ringworm: This is a fungus infection that can affect skin from the scalp (tinea capitis) to the toes (tinea pedis, "athlete's foot"). It is contagious and develops in warm, moist areas of the skin. Obviously, the skin must be kept scrupulously clean and dry. Fungicidal ointments and lotions help.

Eczema: Eczema is not considered a specific disease. The word can apply to a variety of skin disorders including contact dermatitis, described in "Allergies."

Some of the mild skin problems may respond quickly to simple, common-sense care. If they continue or worsen, see a general physician or dermatologist lest they develop into serious skin disorders. Don't try to treat yourself or delay seeing a doctor if you have any of the following:

Cyst or wen	Generalized itching
Furuncle or carbuncle	Canker sores
Abscess	Multiple blisters
Psoriasis	Oozing from skin
Growing moles	Leathery thickening
Crusty, scaly growths	Patches of inflamed skin
Shiny, slick areas	Skin ulcers or tumors

Any dermatitis or infection that won't respond to simple measures
Burns when underlying tissues are affected
Varicose veins that bleed from simple abrasion of skin
Skin discolorations—brown, purple, red, white, yellow—especially
   when over a bump

Although stress is necessary for an interesting life and for "fight or flight" action when endangered, too much stress can be very harmful to mental and physical health. The amount of stress desirable to function at one's best varies with activities and with individuals. Each person should become aware of his own stress level to balance stimulation and relaxation, to help avoid illness, and to discipline overreaction that causes self-destructive tensions.

What body reactions are caused by too much stress? To what ailments does stress contribute? The direct and indirect results of stress, broadly defined, would make a long list of disorders. Stress affects most of the body's systems and influences many organic diseases. Don't try to hide it from your physician.

Sudden stress can quickly increase blood pressure, heartbeat, blood sugar, stomach acid, glandular action (especially in the production of adrenalin), and tightening of artery walls and can cause profuse perspiration, panting, shaking, loss of appetite, and muscular tension.

Continued or recurring stress is related to hypertension, heart problems, strokes, atherosclerosis, phlebitis, diabetes, ulcers, endocrine disturbances, frequent infections, headaches, insomnia, sexual impotence, skin rash and hives, tuberculosis, depression, mental disturbances, alcoholism, and other disorders.

Among the causes of excess stress:

Anxiety	Noise	Hectic pace
Anger	Heat	Overcrowding
Resentment	Cold	Moving
Jealousy	Fatigue	Upset body rhythms
Frustration	Poisons	Jail term
Failure	Injury, illness	Oversensitivity to criticism
Loss of esteem	Financial worries	Death of a spouse
Perfectionism	Boredom	Divorce or separation
Self-disparagement	Retirement	Job change—up, down, or out

Anxiety is probably the most wasteful emotion. It is a dread of some unknown future possibility that may never occur. It makes one feel uneasy, helpless, unnecessarily stressed. On the other hand, fear relates to a known threat that is at hand and is often tangible. Fear can be a "good" stress that alerts you to jump out of the way of a speeding car and gives you the strength to lift a car from a child under a wheel.

What can you do when too much stress is disturbing you?

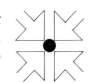

1. If you are already sick or almost sick, tell your physician about your stressful situations. When he is treating your ulcer or hypertension, for instance, he may give you a tranquilizer, suggest how you might cope with anger or problems of retirement, or may recommend a psychiatrist.

2. See people socially. Family and friends soften stressful blows, help restore your sense of values, and motivate you to live the day between yesterday's worries and tomorrow's problems.

3. Let off steam. Laugh. Cry. Walk out to the country and yell. Throw dishes. Hit a tennis or golf ball. Do pushups or any other exercise. Clean cupboards or the garage. For a fresh-start feeling, throw out junk to avoid the urge to throw away gains you have made in your career and personal life.

4. Stresses such as anger and resentment can build up. If not released, the pressure will make something explode, affecting your good health and your good judgment. Talk out your problems to a religious leader, psychiatrist, understanding spouse, friend, or the person reflected in your mirror. Once verbalized, some problems fade or seem smaller and manageable. You gain new perspective.

5. Try to avoid stressful situations. If you cannot, talk to the persons involved, gently but clearly, about what they are doing to your health. Usually the demander, nagger, berater, belittler, money-spender, or noise-maker doesn't realize what he is doing, has no desire to hurt you, is on an "ego trip," or is diverting his own stresses to you because you seem so strong.

6. By nature some people welcome job promotions, new challenges, and extra responsibilities. To others these are stressful. Find out your individual stress levels and set realistic goals. A particular job is not better for you if its demands lead to chronic fatigue, frustration, anxiety, a feeling of underachievement, and ill health.

7. There are "morning" people and "afternoon" people. Assess yourself. Do your most difficult tasks at whatever time you're most energetic and alert. Save easier work for the hours which aren't your prime time.

8. Focus your attention on one main project at a time or you will feel pulled in many directions, causing stress, wasting energy, and depriving you of pleasure in a job well done.

9. If you cannot add more activities to your life without feeling harassed and stressed, learn to say "No" to requests to do favors for friends, committee work, or additional work on your job. You

won't receive any thanks if your performance does not meet expectations, even though the extra work may have been a strain on you.

10. Alternate times of creative, constructive stress when you think and work your best with times of relaxation when you replenish your supply of energy. Train yourself to relax for short periods during a long siege of work. Sit on a straight chair or lie on the floor or other hard surface, close your eyes, and let your muscles go limp. Do a countdown on muscle groups from head to feet (or vice versa), directing each set of muscles to relax, or concentrate on your breathing, mentally repeating some positive word or two with each breath.

11. Stay flexible to changes, a major cause of stress. Bend like a branch in the wind or you will be broken. Adapt to changes in people, procedures, and environment. Why try to fight what you cannot maintain in its present status? Children will grow up and leave home, friends will move or die and new friends will be made, technology and personnel will change at work.

12. Where you can exercise control, plan to space out necessary changes. Each change causes some stress, and a large number at the same time can have a cumulative impact that harms your health. Marrying, traveling in foreign countries for a honeymoon, adjusting to each other, moving to another city, selecting a home and its furnishings, and starting a new job—all within a month—can overwhelm you with stresses. Probably the only reasons some couples come through all right are that they are young enough to stay keyed up for a while and the stresses are excitingly pleasant. People frequently become ill when simultaneous stress situations are the opposite: divorce at middle age, breaking up a familiar home, dividing children and possessions, and losing a job.

13. If you let yourself get angry when driving in snarled traffic or reading a newspaper article on another crisis or stupid error, you are just hurting yourself. Teach yourself to be more patient and tolerant for your health's sake.

14. What is a "good" stress, pleasant and stimulating to some people, may be a "bad" stress to you. Many like loud music or living high in an apartment building; others do not. Attitudes, phobias, and previous experiences play roles in determining stressful situations. When you understand your individual reactions, you can do a great deal to control stress and your health.

Most of this information is to help you have healthy trips abroad. Portions will apply to travel in this country for situations ranging from lost prescriptions to drinking water while camping.

For current information on the immunizations required or recommended for the foreign countries you plan to visit, check with your nearest U.S. Public Health Service (listed in major city phone directories) or the U.S. Center for Disease Control, Atlanta, Georgia 30333 (phone: [404]-633-3311).

Smallpox vaccinations are no longer required by most countries, including the United States. However, if you travel in a country where smallpox still exists or if cases occur in any country within fourteen days of your departure, you must show certified proof of vaccination during the previous three years.

See your physician, preferably two months before departure, for a physical checkup and to check on the following:

1. Inoculations needed. Why leave with a sore arm? Typhoid and paratyphoid immunizations, for instance, require three shots at intervals of seven to ten days. Typhus, tetanus, smallpox, yellow fever, plague, and cholera are on the agenda if you travel to some parts of the world. Ask your physician whether you should also have protection against infectious hepatitis, polio, malaria, or other diseases you may encounter. All of this need not be an ordeal. Some vaccines are combined. You may need only "boosters." But do allow time. A few vaccines may not be available where you live.

   Your doctor enters inoculations on your International Certificate, which must then be certified by your local board of health. Always keep the yellow certificate with your passport. You must show it when entering and leaving each country. And you don't want to lose it between trips abroad.

2. Ask your doctor for typed duplicate prescriptions (to be filled if your luggage is lost) with trade and generic names for any medicines you may be taking. Drug strength is given in the metric system, used internationally. If the medication is made in different types, as for long- or short-term effect, have it specified.

   Carry these reserve prescriptions separately from the medicines you take along. Most American pharmaceuticals are available in the frequently traveled-in countries. Be wary of unknown medications. In a few countries you can buy powerful drugs legally without prescription, but you may endanger your health and life.

3. Ask your doctor whether you should take along antibiotic pills and salve, to be used if necessary.
4. Have the pharmacist completely identify your prescription drugs and take his labeled bottles with you to facilitate Customs inspections.
5. If you have a heart problem, take a recent copy of your electrocardiogram. Ask your doctor to record pertinent data on any disorder you may have, in this book or on a supplemental sheet, in case you need a doctor's care elsewhere.
6. Lack of communication with a foreign physician could be a serious problem. Most hotels and motels have physicians on call, but all do not know the English language. For the names of English-speaking doctors, phone the American Embassy or Consulate in large cities abroad or get a directory by joining the International Association for Medical Assistance to Travelers, Empire State Building, New York, N.Y. 10001. Membership is free; the association is supported by voluntary donations.
7. If you wear a pacemaker or an orthopedic device made with metal such as hip joints or back braces, the metal detectors at airports will sound alarms. To avoid embarrassment and body searches, carry a doctor's letter to show the security guards.
8. If you need an identification bracelet or neck tag for allergies or chronic disorders, always wear it.
9. When going to an area where water and the sanitary growing and handling of food are questionable, ask your doctor for a prescription for the diarrheal problem variously called amebiasis, amebic dysentary, enteric infection, Turista, Montezuma's Revenge, Delhi Belly, Turkey Trots, or Hong Kong Dog. Write down the doctor's directions on dosage and timing.
10. Learn how to protect yourself from communicable diseases wherever sanitary measures do not meet the standards to which your body is accustomed.
    a. Water for drinking and brushing teeth can be purified with nonprescription chlorine tablets. Or order bottled water and make sure the bottle is sealed when you receive it; some hotel employees refill bottles from the tap.
    b. Before eating, wash your hands extra well with soap or use foil-wrapped cleansing towelettes.
    c. Eat raw only the fruits and vegetables you can peel and that have unbroken rinds or skins. Eat oranges instead of ordering orange juice. In some countries oil from the unsanitary rind is also extracted. You can't depend on getting canned fruits and

juices. If you ask for tomato juice, you may be told, "The fruit of the tomato is not yet ripe."

d. Eat food immediately after it has been cooked because bacteria multiply quickly when food stands at room temperature. If at all possible, eat when the dining room of a better hotel or a guidebook-recommended restaurant opens for that mealtime. Otherwise choose a clean-looking, fly-free restaurant. Its hygienic standards are likely to extend to the kitchen. When in doubt, take your antidiarrheal medication. In some restaurants you may feel safer by having simple, well-cooked foods prepared to your order. You may have to wait, but there's less chance for contamination. For the outdoor buffets popular in the tropics, be an early bird in line and touch the outside of the container to make sure the hot dishes are hot and cold ones are cold. Avoid foods that look like leftovers; refrigeration is not dependable. Avoid filled and fancy pastries or hors d'oeuvres; they have been much handled and are usually left at room temperature for hours. Meat, fish, and poultry should be hot and thoroughly cooked. Shun rare steaks, ground meats, and animal organ meats. Where waters appear polluted, don't risk having clams or oysters. Except when there's an outbreak of infectious hepatitis, shrimp, crab, and lobster are generally safe. You're gambling if you eat ice cream, cream, butter, and locally produced cheese in the tropics. Bread is all right unless contaminated by handling or by insects. If in doubt, don't eat the crust.

e. Beverages. Coffee and tea made with local water are safe if the water is freshly boiled. The water content and bottling procedures of American-franchised soft drinks are controlled, but do not use ice which is made from tap water. Beer and alcoholic beverages without ice or tap water are ordinarily safe. If you must have milk, mix the powdered form in chlorinated, boiled, or bottled water in your room. Even where pasteurized, milk may be contaminated by diluting it.

f. Diet if the tourist diarrhea does hit you: Lots of hot tea to replace fluid loss. Plain boiled rice, potatoes, and carrots when nausea stops. Some people like ginger ale (no ice), applesauce, or chewing on cloves. Your nose, taste, and stomach will help guide you when recuperating. Fresh fruit may have a laxative action—which you won't want for a while—but papaya and pineapple contain enzymes, and some find they help to normalize an upset digestive system.

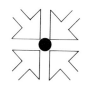

Phone your family doctor, or have someone call for you, as soon as you realize you will need medical attention. If you have been ill all day, why wait until 5 P.M. to call? When a patient is uncooperative, it is unreasonable to expect all-out cooperation from the doctor. He is more likely to say, "Take two aspirin and call me in the morning."

An earlier phone call would enable your doctor to rearrange his schedule to see you that day if prompt examination and a precise diagnosis seem necessary. In the case of a prevalent virus infection or a minor ailment you have had before, the doctor may be able to order treatment by phone.

First tell your doctor the most distressing symptom, such as high fever or abdominal pain; then mention others in descending order of importance. If you have a digestive disturbance, possibly from tainted food, tell the doctor what you ate that might have caused it, when each symptom (nausea, vomiting, or diarrhea) started, and what you have done so far.

If your doctor is not in the office when you phone, tell your major symptoms to his nurse or secretary, who will locate the doctor to return your call. If your call goes to a telephone answering service and your physician is out of town, you will be put in touch with another doctor. In an emergency when your doctor is not immediately available, bypass delays and phone the fire or police department for an ambulance to take you or the sick person to the hospital.

Physicians rarely make house calls nowadays because of travel time and absence of the diagnostic aids which are available in their offices and in hospitals. If you do arrange for a house call, tell the doctor exactly how to reach your home and have someone prepare what the doctor will want.

1. Have warm water, soap, and towel to wash his hands.
2. Have a good light so the patient can really be seen.
3. Provide a straight chair at the bedside.
4. Have table space covered with a clean towel for medical supplies.
5. Have a wastebasket for wrappers, gauze pads, tongue depressor.
6. Keep any other children and pets out of the sickroom.
7. Permit private conversation between doctor and adult patient.
8. Occasionally a place outside of the patient's hearing range is desirable for the doctor to talk with certain members of the family.

If the patient is to remain at home, write down the doctor's directions for medications and other care. Whether you are a weak, feverish patient caring for yourself and sleeping intermittently or a distraught parent caring for a sick child, you are not at peak efficiency. Keep a note pad next to the clock at the bedside. Don't rely on memory, especially when one medication is to be taken every four hours and another every six hours. Jot down the time each medicine is taken.

In taking temperature make sure the thermometer has been shaken down since the last reading, then keep it under the patient's tongue for at least three minutes. Make notes of the temperature and time at every checking. The ups and downs of fever at various times may give the doctor clues to the nature of an infection. Some infections may require laboratory cultures to identify specific bacteria, enabling the doctor to prescribe specific antibiotics.

Do not self-medicate after you have put yourself in the care of a doctor. If you feel you need aspirin, antacids, antidiarrheals, laxatives, sedatives, or anything else that might be in your medicine cabinet, check first with your doctor. The item may be taboo at this time or may be incompatible with the medicine prescribed for this illness. Follow any directions the doctor gives for using moist or dry heat, cold compresses or ice packs, diet, drinking plenty of liquids, or whatever.

When bed rest is ordered, enjoy it. Why prolong an illness by trying to catch up on chores around the house? Make the bed as comfortable as possible, with the lower sheet tight and smooth. Pillows or rolled-up blankets can raise the top sheet and blankets to give toe room when the patient is lying on his back and can serve as a footrest to keep from sliding down when partially sitting up in bed. A backrest can be made with several pillows or anything that forms a wedge shape. A pillow or blanket roll under the knees is also comfortable when the back is at an angle, but don't use it too long lest it hamper circulation to the legs.

If you are caring for a child with a contagious disease, isolate that child from other members of the family, pets, and visitors. They may not be susceptible to the disease but could carry the germs to someone who is. Keep a coverall gown or housecoat in the sickroom, put it on when you enter, and remove it as you leave. Wash hands thoroughly before and after going to the sickroom.

Use disposable paper for dishes and for as many other purposes as possible to avoid the need to use boiling water or disinfectant. Tissues and paper towels have many uses. Disposable sheets and nurse's gowns are available. Anything that cannot be laundered, such as stuffed toys or mattresses, should be aired in the sun after a communicable disease.

Enter a child's infectious disease in his record book to show immunity when the particular disease builds it. A few other childhood disorders may affect later health, and it is important for later doctors to know about them, too.

Put within reach of a bedridden patient a noisemaker to get attention when you are at a distance. A bell or pan to be struck will do. Pin a paper or plastic bag to one side of the bed for soiled tissues and keep a vomit container handy if necessary. Be sure there are no drafts and the air is not too dry in the sickroom. A humidifier, vaporizer, or pan of water on the radiator will add moisture to dry air.

For long-term care in the home, rent a hospital bed. Not only is it more convenient for the patient, but it will save back strain for you when changing linens and sponge-bathing or massaging the patient. If the patient is helpless, he should be turned in bed every three to four hours to avoid bedsores. You can learn this and other techniques from a nurse or by taking a home nursing course offered by the Red Cross.

Children and many elderly people who require prolonged care are usually happier at home than in a hospital or nursing home. If the doctor decides home health care is desirable or needed, he will arrange for visiting nurses or therapists. Medicare and some commercial health insurance policies help pay the cost.

These Doctors Care for Me

For your reference and for doctors who wish to confer with others treating you, give name and phone number on one line. When you move or change doctors in any specialty, draw a fine line through the previous name but do not obliterate it. A former doctor may have valuable data on your health.

Family physician, general practitioner, or internist

_____

_____

_____

_____

_____

_____

_____

_____

Surgeon _____

_____

_____

_____

Pediatrician _____

_____

Allergist _____

_____

Cardiologist _____

_____

General dentist _____

_____

_____

_____

_____

Ophthalmologist, oculist _____

_____

_____

_____

Gynecologist, obstetrician _____

_____

_____

Orthopedist _____

_____

_____

Osteopath _____

_____

Podiatrist, chiropodist _____

_____

Note the specialty, name, and phone number of each additional specialist you might see, e.g., gastroenterologist, endocrinologist, hematologist, neurologist, psychiatrist, dermatologist, proctologist, urologist, chiropractor, otolaryngologist (nose and throat), otologist (ears), oral surgeon, orthodontist, periodontist, endodontist, prosthodontist, geriatrician, and others:

_____

_____

_____

_____

_____

_____

_____

_____

_____

_____

_____

_____

_____

Group plans through employers, labor unions, or affiliations are custom-made to fulfill the needs of the majority in each group. Although a group policy may not meet your own needs exactly, it is more economical than individual coverage. For more coverage, you can supplement it with another policy.

If you are shopping around for a supplemental policy or an individual policy that best meets your situation, you will find a great many differences in policies of the 1,000 companies offering health insurance and in the types issued by a single company.

Consult a trustworthy broker who specializes in the health insurance policies of many companies to select the one that most nearly matches your needs after you have analyzed them. Otherwise, conduct your own investigation to get the most insurance at the lowest cost. You will want good coverage for your most likely expenses and should not have to pay for provisions that might never pertain to you. It is rarely true that the more you pay in premiums, the higher your benefits will be in case of illness or accident.

First check on the financial stability of the companies you are considering. Why entrust your peace of mind and premium payments to a company that may fail before you can collect any benefits due you? Check at least two years' editions of *Best's Insurance Reports* (in large libraries) to find out whether ratings are going up or down. Select a company in one of the two highest *Best's* ratings. If you do not have access to the $90 tome with 1,800 pages, some insurance companies supply small summary reprints.

Next, ask around. Doctors and policy-holding friends can tell you whether they have had problems with certain companies not honoring claims. Write your State Insurance Department or Better Business Bureau to find out whether complaints have been made against the companies.

Commercial insurance companies seldom write policies on any service paid by government agencies: Workmen's Compensation, Employers' Liability Acts, Occupational Disease Laws; for those in the Armed Forces, Veterans' Administration or other federal hospitals, or in tuberculosis or mental hospitals funded by state governments. There are a few disability income plans that will supplement work-related disability benefits, and other policies that offer lump sums for accidental loss of limbs or eyesight or daily benefits for covered accidents while one is in a hospital.

Avoid duplicate coverage. You would just be paying more for no additional benefits. Years ago it was occasionally possible to "make money" on a hospital stay by having policies with two different insurance companies—one paying the hospital and doctor directly, the other sending checks to you. It is no longer possible to receive more than the full cost of medical expenses. Insurance companies require verified copies of itemized medical bills, and they determine which is the primary or subsidiary insurer. To coordinate benefits, codes are used on hospital and doctors' bills.

Types of policies are constantly changing, and some vary with state laws. Coverage obtained also differs with policies described as general, limited, comprehensive, basic, or major medical. One important comparison to consider is this: Indemnity policies provide a flat fee for each day in a hospital, for specific surgical procedures, for a physician's care usually only when hospitalized, and for other items according to the schedule. Premiums are lower, but stated fees rarely cover costs. Service policies offer benefits that pay the total or a percentage of the costs, whatever they may be at the time.

Ordinarily, a basic hospital plan covers the cost of a semiprivate room, board, general hospital services, and routine nursing care. Basic-with-medical coverage adds doctors' visits, in and out of the hospital, and emergency room costs. If surgical care is included, the surgeon's and anesthetist's fees, as well as use of the operating room, are paid. A provision for maternity care is optional.

Major medical insurance supplements basic care with services that may include (depending on the specific plan) inpatient and outpatient diagnostic tests, medications, blood and other intravenous solutions, use of kidney dialysis and other equipment, psychiatry, treatment for mental illness, nursing home care, or other benefits. Major medical plans usually have a deductible anywhere from $50 to $500 of a year's first medical expenses, then pay around 80 percent of further costs up to the policy's limit.

It is prudent to read your policy carefully to find out exactly what is or is not covered. If you do not understand the legal terminology, ask your group administrator or insurance agent for simple, understandable explanations and record them. When you are sick, you will not feel like trying to interpret the sea of fine print on your policy, and you won't want a hassle with the insurer about denied claims while you are recuperating.

Study any "preexisting condition" clauses. Treatment may be excluded for any disorder traceable to an injury or illness sustained while in the Armed Forces. Exclusions for women may be any disorders in the reproductive system. Weigh the advantages of investing your money versus paying premiums for income protection or for disability or catastrophic illness policies.

Analyze your needs. Are your savings sufficient to pay for whatever is not covered in your present policy? Are low-cost clinics available to you? Does your family's health history show serious diseases that may be inheritable? Are you exposed to many risks? Will someone in your family need nursing-home care or extensive dental care?

Many people have too much or too little health insurance or policies not right for them. Here's a checklist to note in various-colored pencils what protection you now have from one or more policies and what you think you may need. These records also offer quick reference when a need for medical care occurs.

Analysis of Health Insurance

Present coverage:

1. Through employer: premiums fully paid _____ or deducted from my pay $ _____ per (period of time) _____ .
2. Through affiliated group: premiums of $ _____ per _____ .
3. Individual membership: premiums of $ _____ per _____ .

No single policy will cover all benefits available; the premiums would be exorbitant. This checklist is to help analyze a present policy or needs for a supplemental or new policy.

1. Policy covers me only _____ , or husband and wife _____ , or one parent and children _____ , or both parents and all children _____ . It covers dependent children up to age _____ with full benefits _____ or _____% of benefits available to husband and wife.
2. Policy starts payments with the first medical bill: Yes _____ . No _____ . If not, deductible at beginning of year is $ _____ and _____% is paid thereafter. Maximum allowed during a year is $ _____ . If not needed one year, can allowances be carried over to the next year? Yes _____ . No _____ .
3. If deductible applies to benefit periods (as in Medicare and some other policies): number of days in a benefit period _____ or _____ days that you can be out of a hospital or nursing home and return for additional care without having another deductible. Are unused reserve days usable later? Yes _____ . No _____ .
4. Hospital inpatient services
   a. Routine nursing care, room, and board allowance: Full

_____or limited to $ _____ per day. Limit of _____ days per illness or admission _____ or per year _____ . In private room _____ , semiprivate room _____ , or ward _____ .

b. Provisions for: Coronary or intensive care unit _____ .

Self-care unit _____ .

Extended care unit (Nursing home) _____ .

c. In any hospital in the world _____ or limited to _____ .

d. Miscellaneous hospital fees: No limit _____ . Limited to $ _____ or _____ % of cost for operating room, X rays, laboratory and other diagnostic tests, medicines, casts, dressings.

5. Hospital outpatient services

a. Emergency first aid: No limit _____ . Limited to $ _____ or _____% per visit _____ or per year _____ .

b. Outpatient diagnostic tests: _____

c. Outpatient elective surgery: _____

6. Surgeons' fees: No limit _____ . Limited to $ _____ or _____ % per year, or limited to amounts in schedule on the policy for each type of operation _____ .

7. Anesthetists' fees: No limit _____ . Limited to $_____ or _____ % per operation.

8. Physicians' fees: No limit _____ . Limited to $ _____ or _____ % or to number of doctors' visits _____ . In-hospital visits only _____ or also office visits and house calls _____ .

9. Ambulance service: No limit _____ . Limited to $ _____ or _____% per year, or limited to one trip to the hospital _____ .

10. Obstetrical service, if the policy includes maternity provisions:

a. For mother: No limit on costs for prenatal, in-hospital, and postnatal care _____ or limited to $ _____ or _____ % of all costs.

b. For baby: Care, including possible need to correct birth defects, from moment of birth _____ or from _____ days after birth. No limit _____ . Limited to $ _____ or _____ % of costs.

11. Waiting time after effective date on policy for coverage of accidents _____ , new illness _____ , preexisting condition (old health problem) _____ , maternity care _____ .

12. Allowances for any prolonged illness _____ .

13. Rehabilitation therapy after strokes or accidents _____ .
14. Are any expenses covered for a voluntary donor of a transplant (skin, cornea, kidney, etc.)? _____ .
15. Is the policy guaranteed renewable (noncancelable by the insurance company)? _____ . Or is it renewable at the option of the insurer? _____ .

In the following, ____ colored pencil checks coverage I have in a present policy and _____ shows coverage I would like:

1. Basic dental care: oral examinations, X rays, cleaning and polishing teeth, amalgam fillings, plastic restorations, topical fluoride applications to children, denture repair, endodontics, simple extractions, and palliative emergency treatment _____ . Basic dental care policies may be extended to include more complex procedures and orthodontics (straightening of teeth) _____ or periodontics (for gum disease) _____ or prosthodontics (bridges and dentures) _____ . A family dental policy may have $25 or $50 deductible per person for the first three members only, then pay 80% of additional dental bills for the year.

2. Medicare supplemental policies to cover expenses not paid by Part A (hospital) or Part B (doctors) _____ .

3. Coverage is also available for:

Convalescent care _____	Physiotherapy _____
Home health services _____	Orthopedic surgery _____
Osteopathic treatments ____	Cosmetic surgery _____
Psychiatry _____	Drug addiction _____
Psychotherapy _____	Elective abortion _____
Sterilization _____	

   Chiropractic treatments (covered in 35 states) _____
   Mental disorders where states do not cover _____
   Alcoholism (required by most states in all general policies, but some are limited to inpatient care) _____
   Extra household and living expenses when convalescing or an invalid _____
   Disability income of $_____ per month or _____ % of pay
   If permanent disability, you may be eligible for Social Security.

4. Other benefits wanted _____

_____ .

116

My Health Insurance Policies

(Keep this section up to date.)

Insurance Co. _____

Employer/Group _____

Family member's name _____

Insurance Co. _____

Employer/Group _____

Family member's name _____

Insurance Co. _____

Employer/Group _____

Family member's name _____

Insurance Co. _____

Employer/Group _____

Family member's name _____

Insurance Co. _____

Employer/Group _____

Family member's name _____

Insurance Co. _____

Employer/Group _____

Family member's name _____

Insurance Co. _____

Employer/Group _____

Family member's name _____

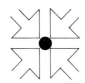

When a doctor is not present and a few minutes' delay could mean death or severe damage to a person's health, rescue may depend on you alone or on you as part of a team. Here are some ways you could save a family member or a friend or be a good samaritan to a stranger.

If you see a person who is unconscious for no apparent reason, look for an identification bracelet, neck tag, or wallet card (described in "Checkpoints to Guard Your Health"). It could tell you of a health problem that needs immediate medical attention.

Learn how to give CPR (cardiopulmonary resuscitation), mouth-to-mouth breathing and rhythmic chest compression. CPR is needed immediately in cardiac arrest, drowning, suffocation, strangulation, barbiturate overdosage, and carbon monoxide inhalation. Practice on a dummy mannequin, not on a living person, until you have the ability to perform CPR correctly. In various areas instruction is given by Civil Defense Units, the Red Cross, fire departments, hospitals, schools, or the American Heart Association.

When a person collapses while eating, first make sure it is not a heart attack by asking, "Can you talk?" If the person shakes his head "No," there is probably a chunk of food (bolus) stuck in the windpipe. It must be removed in less than five minutes or the person will die from food asphyxiation.

One way to remove the food obstruction is called the Heimlich maneuver. Stand behind the person and put both arms around his waist, letting the person's head, arms, and upper torso hang forward. Make a fist with one of your hands and grasp that wrist with your other hand. Press the fist forcefully into his upper abdomen with a quick upward thrust. Repeat several times. This pushes up the diaphragm, compresses air in the lungs, and makes the bolus in the air passage pop out. If you choke on food while alone, simulate this action with your own fist or hang over a corner of a heavy chair to apply force just below the diaphragm.

Another technique is to use the curved plastic tweezers most restaurants have to retrieve a bolus. If not immediately at hand, lay the person on his side, give one quick whack between the shoulder blades, open the person's mouth, and with your fingers pull out the obstructing food. This is no time for niceties or sanitary measures. An average of six people a day in the United States choke to death with "cafe coronaries," so-called because they frequently happen when drinking, laughing, and eating with friends at cafes.

The United States government has designated certain hospitals to be Poison Control Centers. Usually one large hospital serves a multi-city area, but in a few large cities a children's hospital has also been named. The Poison Control Centers keep up-to-date data on toxic ingredients in specific medicines, insecticides, and household and commercial products, and have facts on plants.

If a poison was swallowed, note the plant or flower eaten or grab the product container and dial Operator for the nearest Poison Control Center. Better yet, find out now what hospital the Poison Control Center is in and note name, address, and phone: _____

_____ .

You will be told what to do immediately. Don't guess. If the person is unconscious, has swallowed a corrosive or petroleum product, or has a burning pain in mouth or throat, do not induce vomiting. Get instructions. Antidotes for poisons vary. For some you may be told to induce vomiting by tickling the back of the throat or by having the person drink warm water with mustard powder, salt, or vinegar—then keeping his or her head lower than the hips so vomitus cannot enter the lungs. Antidotes for other toxic substances may be milk, baking soda, mineral oil, egg white, milk of magnesia, tea, or medicinal charcoal. Especially if you have children, keep activated charcoal on hand; it absorbs many poisons. When the poisonous substance is not known, rush the person to a hospital for blood tests to find out.

Often the correct immediate measure for swallowed poisons is sufficient. If further care is needed, take the person to the Poison Control Center. Where too distant, it will give information to your nearest hospital, clinic, or doctor. First care for skin burns from heat or chemicals is lots of cold water.

In an accident, if broken bones or internal injuries are suspected, don't move the person unless absolutely necessary to save him or her from further harm. In that case move the body lengthwise, with all parts supported on a blanket, long coat, door, or wide board. If certain that only an arm or leg is broken, pad it with clothing, support it with temporary splints made from skis or boards, then wrap snugly. If at all possible, wait for medical aid. To lessen shock, loosen tight clothing, keep the person warm but not perspiring, and give assurance in a calm tone.

In cases with severe bleeding, help the person lie down to prevent fainting. With your whole hand, firmly press over the wound a sterile bandage or the cleanest cloth available. Learn the four pressure points to control arterial blood supply to arms and legs. Let the doctor clean and treat wide or deep wounds.

For fainting, place the person on his back with the head lower than the rest of the body if possible. Loosen tight clothing. Apply cold wet cloths to his or her face and forehead. Do *not* slap the face, shake the person, or expect an unconscious person to drink water. If the fainter does not revive in two minutes, take him to a hospital emergency room or phone for an ambulance. Fainting may be caused by fatigue, heat, hunger, or a poorly ventilated room—or it may be a symptom of diabetic coma, insulin reaction, alcohol and barbiturate coma, or other problem that needs prompt medical attention.

Electric shock is another emergency situation that won't wait for a doctor. Break contact with the source of electricity the quickest, safest way. Disconnect the plug of the faulty appliance, protecting yourself by handling it with dry rubber gloves or through several layers of dry, heavy fabric; or pull the main switch at the fuse box. If the body is touching a fallen live wire outside, remove the body from contact, using a dry pole, branch, rope, or clothing—no metal. Stand in a dry place and do not touch the person until contact is broken. Then, if necessary, use CPR and phone for medical assistance.

Study first-aid guides until you are thoroughly familiar with all procedures. You won't have time to read them in real emergencies. Keep first-aid kits at home and in your car. Check them occasionally to make sure the antiseptic hasn't leaked out and that gauze pads and adhesive or plastic strips are still sterile in unbroken individual wraps.

The fastest way to get experienced help to the scene of an accident, stroke, heart attack, childbirth, or other reason for immediate hospitalization and care en route is to phone for an ambulance with trained attendants. In a few localities this may be a hospital ambulance with intern or nurse, but usually it is a fire or police department ambulance with paramedics or EMTs (emergency medical technicians).

They hook the patient up to a telemetric system that electronically measures pulse, respiration, and blood pressure, recording them, and recording electrocardiograms as well, in a hospital. Or the paramedics take vital signs and tell them to a doctor in a hospital miles away with two-way radio communication. A doctor gives directions for defibrillation (shock to normalize heartbeat), intravenous solutions, or other care to revitalize or stabilize a patient before and during the ride to the hospital emergency room. For an ambulance

with trained personnel in your area, phone _____.

Find out where Trauma Centers are located in your community. They are staffed and equipped to give emergency care all day and night. Blue-and-white signs before exits from highways direct motorists to them, but it is advisable to know those closest to your home and along frequently traveled routes. List Trauma Centers here:

_____

_____

_____

Because emergency rooms are frequently operated at a loss, hospitals in many large cities have developed cooperative programs. A hospital in the *comprehensive* category has a physician in the emergency room at all times, every type of specialist on call, and a radiologist and laboratory technicians on staff day and night. A *basic* hospital has a physician on duty at all times and specialists in surgery, pediatrics, and maternity care, as well as auxiliary personnel, on call. A *standby* hospital has a registered nurse on duty and a physician on call to give emergency service.

Comprehensive hospital: _____

Address _____ **Phone** _____

Basic hospital: _____

Address _____ **Phone** _____

Standby hospital: _____

Address _____ **Phone** _____

Blood Donations

Blood is (or should be) taken only from healthy individuals, without danger to them or to those to whom it will be given. During wartime it was found that giving blood acted as a tonic to the donor, stimulating the bone marrow to replenish the blood faster after each donation—just as physical exercise stimulates muscles. The pint of blood given is replaced by the body in around a month.

In many areas blood banks are set up by groups. Members donate blood on regular schedules, increasing donations when there are emergencies. As needed, members and their families can have free transfusions. If not in a group that provides this service, as an individual you may donate one or two pints a year and receive prorated benefits for you and your family. Some hospitals will also take your blood a month or so before elective surgery and give your own blood back to you in a transfusion after surgery.

Blood is collected, processed, and stored in a center or in individual hospitals which have a cooperative blood replacement program. If the blood was not pretested, it is checked for viral hepatitis and syphilis, and it is categorized as A, B, O, AB, Rh negative or positive, or rare blood type.

Because blood components rather than whole blood are used to treat many diseases, blood for storage is spun in a centrifuge to separate it. Plasma, a yellowish fluid, is frozen and will keep for around a year. Platelets to clot blood must be used within three days. White cells to fight infections are effective for only six hours, but red cells which transport oxygen have a longer life. Whole blood is frozen, but the process is more expensive and used mainly for rare blood types and for transfusions to the individual who gave it prior to surgery.

One out of every fourteen hospitalized patients needs some component of blood or whole blood. Over 6 million transfusions are given each year. The acceptability of your blood for a donation is determined by a drop or two taken from an earlobe or fingertip. As for general requirements, you can be a donor if you:

1. Are a healthy adult between eighteen and sixty-five years old.
2. Do not weigh less than 110 pounds (50 kilograms) if a woman or 125 pounds (56.7 kilograms) if a man.
3. Have not given blood in the previous eight weeks. Some organizations specify six months between donations.
4. Have not had tuberculosis, diabetes, viral hepatitis, or syphilis. Former malaria patients may now donate three years after recovery.

5. Have not had a severe cold, sore throat, acute allergy, or attack of hay fever, asthma, or hives in the previous two weeks.
6. Are not taking drugs, except tranquilizers or birth-control pills.
7. Have not had major surgery in six months or a tooth extraction in the last two weeks.
8. Are not pregnant and have not been during the last six months.
9. Do not have high or low blood pressure.
10. Are not fatigued at the time of giving blood.
11. Have not had any immunizations in the last two weeks.
12. Will not have any alcohol within twelve hours before donating and will eat only a light meal around four hours before donating.

When and Where I've Donated Blood

Date	Place (hospital, organization with mobile unit, other)

Medical science is working on ways to avoid rejections of transplants without the use of powerful immunosuppressive drugs which reduce the recipient's ability to fight infection. It is hoped that eventually *almost* any defective, severely injured, or worn-out part of a body may be replaced. Advance treatments given to patients or to the organs have made it possible to transplant skin, corneas, pancreas cells, and adrenal, thymus, or thyroid glands. The heart-transplant situation has not yet been resolved.

Kidney transplants have been the most successful to date, especially when the persons are closely related. Donor and recipient can live with one kidney each. Bone marrow transplants have achieved some success when tissues of both individuals are matched. The hospital will give you and the recipient careful medical examinations and supply the consent forms.

If you are over eighteen and wish to donate your body or any organs or parts, if medically acceptable, to take effect upon your death, you can get a wallet-sized Uniform Donor Card from the Kidney Foundation. Look under "K" for this name in the phonebook of any large city to find the address of the regional office nearest you. If you live in a small city or town, write to National Kidney Foundation, 116 East 27th Street, New York, N.Y. 10016. The headquarters will forward your request to your regional office which will mail you the requested number of cards for adults in your family.

Always carry the card, (copy shown at right), in your wallet. In case of accidental death, it will inform a doctor or hospital of your wishes. Your family will be called for verification, so tell adult members. Expressing your wishes in your Will is of no value. That document won't be read until it is too late for your gift of an organ to be of use to anyone else. Consult your physician for further information.

UNIFORM DONOR CARD

OF _____
Print or type name of donor

In the hope that I may help others, I hereby make this anatomical gift, if medically acceptable, to take effect upon my death. The words and marks below indicate my desires.

I give: (a)——any needed organs or parts
(b)——only the following organs or parts

_____
Specify the organ(s) or part(s)

for the purposes of transplantation, therapy, medical research or education:

(c)——my body for anatomical study if needed.

Limitations, or
special wishes, if any:_____

Signed by the donor and the following two witnesses in the presence of each other:

_____   _____
Signature of Donor   Date of Birth of Donor

_____   _____
Date Signed   City & State

_____   _____
Witness   Witness

This is a legal document under the Uniform Anatomical Gift Act or similar laws.

It is merely annoying to undergo the indignities imposed upon a patient in a hospital for illness, surgery, or diagnostic tests such as proctoscopy. There are short, stiff, scratchy gowns, infusions and transfusions, noises, bedpans, intrusions on privacy.

You will bear temporary discomforts and be grateful for medical technology that helps restore your health even though it might require tubes in body cavities, needles strapped on limbs, a monitor on the heart, an oxygen mask over nose and mouth, drains after surgery, or a link to a kidney dialysis machine.

However, should a terminally ill patient who may prefer to die in peace be forced to accept massive measures merely to sustain a flicker of life for a few more days or months? This is a question with pros and cons being argued by doctors and lawyers.

The American Bar Association in 1975 adopted the standard that death occurs when the brain stops functioning, even though machines are sustaining circulation and respiration. Most doctors agree. The question to be decided is at what point the patient shall be declared legally dead. Harvard University researchers in 1968 suggested that it be when electroencephalograms, taken twenty-four hours apart, show no brain activity. Dead brain cells do not revive.

Since then the National Institute of Neurological Diseases and Stroke conducted a three-year study in nine institutions where doctors determined that, after many additional tests, brain death could be declared in as little as thirty minutes. A standard of less than twenty-four hours could reduce the delay for transplants, if offered, and would save money and emotional trauma for the family.

State legislatures are considering the criteria to be used and proposed laws to permit "death with dignity." These statutes would recognize the rights of terminally ill persons to direct that no extensive artificial methods be used solely to sustain life processes when patients prefer to die naturally.

Many individuals realize they may not be able to decide or make their wishes known when they are terminally ill. While still healthy, they sign a request that death be allowed to occur if or when there would be no hope of restoring even limited ability for living and the laws of their states permit the right to die.

This is a voluntary, thoughtful way of looking toward the future. It helps to relieve relatives and physicians in making agonizing decisions and to avoid drains on family finances. It protects patients from the continuance of intense pain without hope of surcease, the indignities of physical and psychological deterioration, and the dependence on machines to maintain the minimal signs of life.

Death with Dignity

The only professional organization which has adopted and approved a suggested form for a patient's right to die with dignity, as of this writing, is the Connecticut State Medical Society, which has given permission to reprint from its statement entitled "Dignity in Life and Death," approved by the Society's House of Delegates in April of 1973.

To My Family, My Physician, My Clergyman, My Lawyer:

If the time comes when I can no longer actively take part in decisions for my own future, I wish this statement to stand as the testament of my wishes.

If there is no reasonable expectation of my recovery from physical or mental and spiritual disability, I, _____ _____ , request that I be allowed to die and not be kept alive by artificial means or heroic measures. I ask also that drugs be mercifully administered to me for terminal suffering even if in relieving pain they may hasten the moment of death. I value life and the dignity of life, so that I am not asking that my life be directly taken, but that my dying not be unreasonably prolonged, nor the dignity of life destroyed.

This request is made, after careful reflection, while I am in good health and spirits. Although this document is not legally binding, you who care for me will, I hope, feel morally bound to take it into account. I recognize that it places a heavy burden of responsibility upon you, and it is with the intention of sharing this responsibility that this statement is made.

Date _____ **Signed** _____

Witnessed by: _____

_____

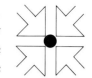

As you find out how the body functions, you will be fascinated, awed, and appreciative of this wondrous, complicated machine. Practically every science and technology is represented in the body. All the experiences your body has ever had and your reactions to them are recorded in the brain, though you may not be aware of them. Introduce your body to your mind. You'll find out you can take more control over maintaining your health than you thought possible.

All over the body, each individual is as unique as his thumbprint. Normal ranges, averages, or medians can be statistically figured, but no one person is ideal in all measurements of health.

Find out your own norms or levels for best functioning and your strong or weak points. Not every part of you is scrutinized often and long enough by professionals. Only you are with your body twenty-four hours a day. You attend to its particular needs for food, water, rest, elimination, temperature control, environmental protection. You sense each pang or ache.

Why not get to know how to interpret the signals your body gives for professional care, too? What symptoms may you safely ignore and what ones need a doctor's attention? For example, excessive thirst and frequent urination are signs of diabetes, yet many fail to recognize them. The U.S. Public Health Service reports half of the estimated 4 million diabetics in the country do not know they have this disease though the urine test is routine in physicians' offices, hospitals frequently publicize free diabetic tests for anyone who walks in, and home-testing strips are available.

There are three ways to diagnose a disease. Doctors say some diseases are determined mainly from a patient's history, others mainly by the physical examination, and a few mainly by diagnostic tests. Most diseases require a combination of all three. Yet surveys made by doctors have shown that the majority of doctors do not take patient histories or take only cursory ones and less than one physician in thirty makes an adequate physical examination. A government agency reports that one quarter of the diagnostic tests made are unreliable.

Doesn't that suggest you had better become involved? Your own health records in this book will be more complete than any doctor's "history" of you. The doctor depends a great deal on what you tell him, so your knowledge of your own body and of symptoms of disorders can help guide the doctor in examining the disturbed area at least. Knowing about diagnostic tests can help you cooperate to increase accuracy and knowing they aren't always reliable may alert you on when to ask for repetitions of tests.

Discover Your Own Body

127

The more you know about your body, the more intelligently you can discuss problems with a doctor. The more information you have on the health care system, the better you will be able to fit into the system for your own benefit. When tests are being made, you must adapt to the system for efficiency reasons, despite lip service given to treating a patient as a person. But if you know what's going on and why, you need not feel like a nonperson throughout the procedures. You can be an interested cooperator and learn much about your health.

When you know, you won't be misled by attendants such as those who told a patient to walk to his bed after an angiogram. You won't accept the word of a doctor who dismisses a treatable condition as simply due to old age. You won't take the word of an office nurse who gives you a date you can return to work without checking with the surgeon. You won't be passive when a doctor says "We'll wait and watch" a lump in a neck for a year before observing, "Well, it's getting bigger now. Maybe we'd better take it out." By that time the malignancy had spread through the twenty-five-year-old man's body. You won't let a doctor dismiss a distressing symptom by saying, "That's not due to the drug," without checking into the reason for the symptom. These and other unfortunate instances have happened to unknowing patients.

In addition to their years of schooling, internship, and practice, doctors are expected to get fifty hours of continuing education each year. Is fifty hours a year, an hour a week, devoted to the study of health too much to expect of patients who do not have the background education and ongoing experience of doctors? Are you regularly reading books and articles on health? Have you taken any courses in health since your school hygiene or physiology classes?

Suggestions have been made that doctors establish programs for patient education to teach patients about their bodies, possible dysfunctions, and health maintenance. But have you ever had a physician teach you the functions of an organ or a system of the body, how a disease in one part can affect others, and what you might do to avoid or lessen problems? Most doctors admit they are treatment-oriented and can't take time to teach prevention of disorders. They give *sick care*, not *health care*.

Then who is responsible for your health care? *You!* It's up to you to know about health, your own body's health, and to keep records in cooperation with your doctors. When you need sick care—what doctors don't know about you can cost money, illness, your life!